Pregnancy and birth

a guide for deaf women

by Sabina Iqbal

Published by RNID in association
with the National Childbirth Trust

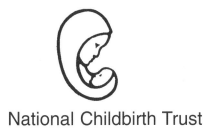

National Childbirth Trust

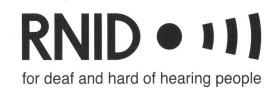

for deaf and hard of hearing people

Published by RNID in association with the National Childbirth Trust.

RNID, 19-23 Featherstone Street, London EC1Y 8SL.
Telephone 0808 808 0123
Textphone 0808 808 9000
Fax 020 7296 8199
E-mail informationline@rnid.org.uk
Website www.rnid.org.uk

Registered Charity No. 207720

The National Childbirth Trust,
Alexandra House, Oldham Terrace,
Acton, London W3 6NH.
Telephone 0870 444 8707
Textphone 020 8993 6714
Fax 0870 770 3237
E-mail enquiries@national-childbirth-trust.co.uk
Website www.nctpregnancyandbabycare.com

Registered Charity No. 801395

To order more copies of this book contact RNID.

ISBN 1 904296 03 3
The photographs in this book have been reproduced with the permission of the following.

Front and Back cover – Philip Meech
[main photographer]
Foreword – Philip Meech
Contents - Philip Meech

1 Philip Meech, 3 Lewis Photos Ltd, 5 Philip Meech 8-9 Lewis Photos Ltd, 10 Lewis Photos Ltd (top), Alex Segre, 11 Philip Meech (top), Lewis Photos Ltd (below), 12 Philip Meech, 14-15 Philip Meech, Page 18-19 Mothercare, 20 Mothercare (top) & Alex Segre (bottom page), 23 Alex Segre (bottom page), 24 Philip Meech (top), 24 Lewis Photos Ltd, 25 – NCT Publishing, 26-27 Philip Meech, 28 Chris Kelly, 29 Alex Segre, 30 Philip Meech (top), Lewis Photos Ltd (below), 31 Lewis Photos Ltd, 32 Crispin Hughes, 33 Alex Segre, 34 Philip Meech (top), Bubbles (below), 35 Philip Meech, 36 Chris Kelly, 39 Science Photo Library, 41 Science Photo Library, 42 Philip Meech, 43 Alex Segre, 44 Philip Meech, 45 Science Photo Library, 47 Lewis Photos Ltd, 48 Chris Kelly, 49 Alex Segre, 50 Philip Meech, 51 Science Photo Library, 52 National Childbirth Trust (NCT), 54 Tracy Grant (top), Alex Segre (bottom), 55 Philip Meech, 57 National Childbirth Trust (NCT) (top), 57 Philip Meech (Bottom), 58 NCT, 59 Science Photo Library (top, right), 59 Mothercare (middle, left), 60 Bubbles Photo Library, 66 Alex Segre, 67 Philip Meech, 68 Science Photo Library, 69 NCT Publishing, 70 Lewis Photos Ltd, 71 NCT Publising, 72 NHS Newborn Hearing Screening Programme (NHSP), 73 as above, 74 as above, Alex Segre (bottom), 75 NCT Publishing, 76 NCT Publishing, 77 Philip Meech, 78 NCT Publishing, 79 NCT Publising, 80 Alex Segre, 81 Philip Meech, 82 BLISS (photographer Paula Glassman), 83 Alex Segre, 84 Philip Meech, 85 Mothercare, 86 The Foundation for the study of Infant Deaths, 87 Philip Meech (top), Alex Segre (bottom), 88 Philip Meech (top), Alex Segre (bottom), 90 Philip Meech (top), Alex Segre (bottom), 91 Philip Meech, 92 Crispin Hughes, 94 Philip Meech, 95 Lewis Photos Ltd, 96 Alex Segre, 97 Philip Meech (top photo), Science Photo Library (main), 98 Alex Segre, 99 Philip Meech, 100 Brian Morrison, 101 Chris Kelly, 102 Brian Morrison, 103 Alex Segre, 108 Philip Meech, 111 Alex Segre, 112 Philip Meech, 117 Alex Segre, 118 Philip Meech, 132 Philip Meech, 134 Lewis Photos Ltd (top), Alex Segre (middle), Philip Meech (bottom).

Illustrations
© 2004 Annabel Milne

Design by Julie Goldsmith RNID
Edited by Gill Kirby

Foreword

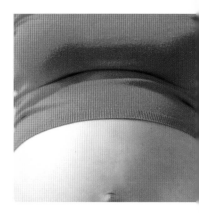

As a deaf mother I found this book clear, heart-warming and fun to read. There is a lot to take in when you're pregnant but the information in this book is easy to read and absorb with lots of pictures, bullet points and tips. All the stories from deaf women make it come alive. When I had my own daughter I found the lack of clear information stressful and would have welcomed a book like this.

I hope all deaf fathers will read the whole book, not just 'their' chapter. I also welcome the section written for health professionals. Clear and supportive communication can help pregnant deaf women when their priority is their baby. I had an induced birth which I found very upsetting – if my doctors had been more deaf aware I would have been able to understand what was going on and would have had a better experience. I recall how important it was for the midwives and doctors to remember to pull down their face masks so that I could lipread them, especially when they were shouting "push"!

As far as I am aware this is the only book published in the UK which has been written solely for deaf mothers, mothers-to-be, and the professionals who work with them. I commend this book to you. Have a jolly good read!

Laraine Callow

Mother of a now grown up daughter and Director of her own company – Deafworks. Deafworks delivers customised packages to voluntary, statutory and commercial organisations and is committed to training and development for the future of D/deaf people and the wider community. Laraine has had a long and successful career in education working with both deaf and hard of hearing parents and their deaf babies and children. She has also been a teacher of English and a teacher of the deaf. She is an experienced trainer and has counselling skills. Laraine has produced many leaflets, factsheets and information guides for deaf people and is currently writing a book.

Contents

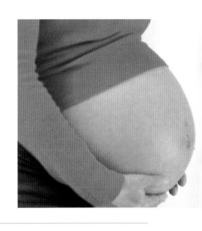

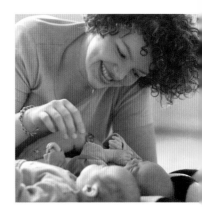

Chapter 1
About this book

Stories from deaf mothers

This book has been written for deaf women so you will find their stories throughout the book. Sabina Iqbal interviewed eight parents in depth – six deaf women, one deafened woman and one deaf man. They all have children under three years old. Each of the interviews was video taped and carried out in either British Sign Language (BSL) or Sign-Supported English (SSE). One mother spoke during her interview. Sabina also used a questionnaire to back up the interviews. Once the interviews were completed she used the video tapes and notes she had taken to write up the stories in the parents' own words. They have been edited as little as possible to ensure that they reflect the true experiences that deaf parents face in accessing services.

In addition, several parents also came forward to share their experiences by e-mail and we have included some of their stories in this book.

All names have been changed in this book.

Deaf fathers

This book is written mainly for deaf mothers and mothers-to-be but we have included some stories from deaf fathers. If you are a deaf father, or a deaf father-to-be, we hope you will find all of this book useful. We have also included a chapter for you.

We would like to thank all those parents who so kindly gave up time to share their stories with Sabina.

Information for health professionals

If you are a health professional working with a pregnant deaf woman or a new deaf parent, we hope you'll read all of this book, but in case you don't have time, or you need a quick reference, we have included a section just for you.

How to use this book

We have divided this book into chapters beginning with planning a baby and ending with information for health professionals.

This book does not cover everything about pregnancy and birth. We have explained key advice and information that deaf mothers and mothers-to-be, are most likely to want to know.

At the end of every section we have suggested other organisations and websites that can give you more information on particular subjects. You could read this book in parts, while looking at one of the many other baby books and magazines you can get easily in bookshops. We have included a list of books and videos that you may find useful.

If you have any worries...

If you have any worries or concerns about your health or your pregnancy you should always contact your GP (family doctor) or midwife. They will be able to tell you if there is nothing wrong, or get you medical attention if it is needed.

Medical words

Because this is a book about pregnancy we have used medical words – from 'amniotic fluid' to 'fallopian tube'. These words are explained when we use them, and we have a glossary at the end of this book. If you come across a word you don't understand, check to see if it's in the glossary. We also use diagrams and photos to help describe what we mean.

Describing your baby

Sometimes in this book you will find us talking about your baby as 'she' or 'her'. We use these words to describe a boy or girl baby as we think this sounds better than 'it'.

Up-to-date information

At the time of going to press all the information in this book is up-to-date and reflects the latest medical advice available. However, advice for pregnant mothers and new mothers can change. You should always ask your midwife or GP for advice if you are unsure about anything you have read.

Describing deafness

Being deaf or hard of hearing can mean very different things to different people. Some people feel more comfortable with particular words to describe their own deafness. You might feel quite strongly about terms that you do not like being used. RNID uses the following terms:

Deaf people. We use the term deaf people in a general way when we are talking about people with all degrees of deafness.

Hard of hearing people. We use the term hard of hearing people to describe people with a mild to severe hearing loss. We quite often use it to describe people who have lost their hearing gradually.

Deafened people. People who were born hearing and became severely or profoundly deaf after learning to speak are often described as deafened.

Deafblind people. Many deafblind people have some hearing and vision. Some are totally deaf and totally blind.

The Deaf Community. Many Deaf people whose first or preferred language is BSL consider themselves part of the Deaf Community. They may describe themselves as 'Deaf', with a capital D, to emphasise their Deaf identity.

We use the term deaf people throughout this book to refer to deaf, deafened and hard of hearing people. We have also used a capital D where individual parents choose to describe themselves in this way.

If you are hearing and would like to find out more about how deaf people communicate, including BSL and lipreading, please see *Chapter 20 Information for health professionals*.

About the writer – Sabina Iqbal (née Chowdry)

Sabina is Asian, Deaf, and a British Sign Language (BSL) user. She is a qualified social worker and worked with Asian Deaf people for a local authority for several years. She is currently a Deaf/Hard of Hearing Services Development Officer for Westminster City Council.

In 2001 she researched deaf parenting in the USA as part of her International Social Work Studies degree. Her research highlighted the barriers many American deaf parents face when they want access to information and services about pregnancy, health and their children's education.

Sabina found services and information for deaf parents in the UK were also poor. In response she helped set up the Deaf Parenting Project. The Project aims to explore ways of improving access to information for deaf parents and parents-to-be.

Since then Sabina has been involved in a number of projects for deaf parents, including:

- A video about deaf parents' experience of pregnancy and the early stages of being a parent called *Deaf parents – Gaps in Services*.
- A Deaf Parenting e-mail group that puts deaf parents, and professionals who work with them, in touch with each other to share information and offer support (see *Chapter 21 Further information*).
- Several workshops and presentations about deaf parenting.
- www.deafparent.org.uk – a website for deaf parents, professionals working with deaf parents and service providers.

Sabina also works as a freelance trainer and consultant on Ethnic Deaf issues. She has also appeared as a reporter/presenter for BBC See Hear, on local council information videos, and as a Deaf interpreter for Signpost, a translation service at Tees-TV.

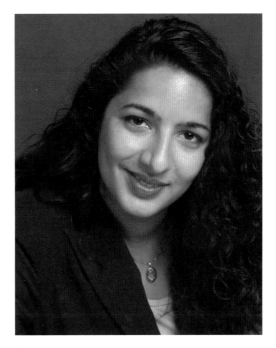

Our advisory panel

We would like to thank the following members of our advisory panel for their helpful advice and comments.

Penny Beschizza, Co-ordinator to Deaf Students, Southwark College
Penny is a Deaf mother of two grown up children. As a college teacher of young deaf adults she is frequently asked for clear, deaf-friendly information her students can use and keep for when they themselves become parents. She is also a BSL tutor, trainer in Deaf Awareness and a member of NATFHE's (the University and College Lecturers' Union) Equality Advisory Committee.

Marije Davidson, Legal Policy Officer, RNID
Marije is a Deaf mother with three children under six. She was born profoundly deaf and grew up in the Netherlands. She has a law degree and has worked as a disability policy officer for the Dutch government. She was also a member of the Government Committee on Sign Language of the Netherlands.

Clare Flory
Clare is Deaf and has worked in the field of disability for several years including the Employers' Forum on Disability, RNID and National Deaf Children's Society.

Juliet Goddard, Postnatal Tutor, National Childbirth Trust
Juliet has a professional background in social work. She is currently working on a project to increase access to information for all parents and their families. Juliet is hearing.

Becki Josiah, Information Officer, Disability Pregnancy Parenthood International (DPPi)
Becki has been involved in the issue of deaf parenting for several years. She has worked closely with Sabina and they both helped set up the Deaf Parenting Project at DPPi. Becki is hearing and her maternal grandparents were Deaf. She is also a mother of two children and a foster parent.

Zita Killick, Senior Lecturer Midwifery, Anglia Polytechnic University
Zita is a qualified midwife and teacher with midwifery, nursing and teaching experience. She studied maternity care for deaf women as part of an MSc in Inter-professional Practice in Health and Social Care. Zita is hearing.

Simon Robinson, Legal Officer, RNID
Simon is a qualified barrister with extensive experience in discrimination law and human rights in both the courts and tribunals. He is a member of the Bar Council Disability Committee. Simon is hearing.

Elaine Seth-Smith
Elaine is an employment solicitor with extensive knowledge of maternity rights and benefits. Elaine is hearing.

Asha Sharma MRCOG, Consultant Obstetrician and Gynaecologist, St John's Hospital, Mid Essex Hospital Trust
Asha is a Member of the Royal College of Obstetricians and Gynaecologists. She is the Director of Obstetric Services and is the lead for risk management within obstetrics at St John's Hospital.

Lynn Waddell, Disability Nurse Specialist, Forth Valley Primary Care NHS Trust
Lynn teaches and supports all health care professionals within the Forth Valley area, including midwives. She is hearing and was brought up within a profoundly Deaf family so has always signed. She is a registered lipspeaker, deafblind communicator and registered CACDP (The Council for the Advancement of Communication with Deaf People) tutor in Deaf Awareness and Communication Tactics.

National Childbirth Trust

We are very pleased to publish this book in association with the National Childbirth Trust – the largest and best-known childbirth and parenting charity in Europe. It offers wide-ranging information and support at UK level and locally, through its 380 branches. The National Childbirth Trust is consulted by decision-makers on all aspects of pregnancy, birth and early parenting and works hard for improved maternity care and better services and facilities for new parents.

We would particularly like to thank Patricia Wise and Cynthia Masters-Waage for their help and advice.

Cynthia Masters-Waage, Antenatal Tutor, National Childbirth Trust
Cynthia works as a counsellor and doula (see *Glossary*), as well as teaching antenatal classes. She has supported deaf women during antenatal and aqua natal classes and during labour and birth. Cynthia is hearing.

Patricia Wise, Breastfeeding Counsellor Tutor, National Childbirth Trust
Patricia was originally a science teacher and has a Diploma in Counselling. She has three children. Patricia is hearing.

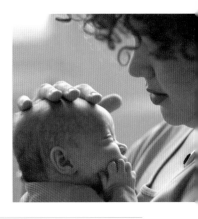

Chapter 2
Planning a baby

Getting help and advice from your Family Planning Clinic

Your local Family Planning Clinic can give you advice about contraception (birth control) and planning a baby. Family Planning Clinics are usually based at your GP surgery, at sexual health clinics or women's health centres. Ask your GP if you want to know where your nearest family planning clinic is.

What sort of support and advice will my GP give me?

GP means 'General Practitioner' and is another word for your local doctor. Your GP can give you advice about planning your pregnancy and can:

- Check your medical notes to see if there is anything about your own health that might affect your baby. If you are taking any medicine talk to your doctor before trying for a baby.
- Give you advice about how your pregnancy can affect your health.
- Carry out any tests you may need, for example, you may be given a blood test for German measles – also known as rubella.

Why is it important to have a rubella vaccination?

It is important because if you get rubella during your pregnancy it can harm your baby. You may have had a rubella vaccination when you were young, but your GP will test you to see whether you need another one. If you do, your GP or nurse will offer you another vaccination. If you are given the rubella vaccination, you must wait over three months before trying for a baby.

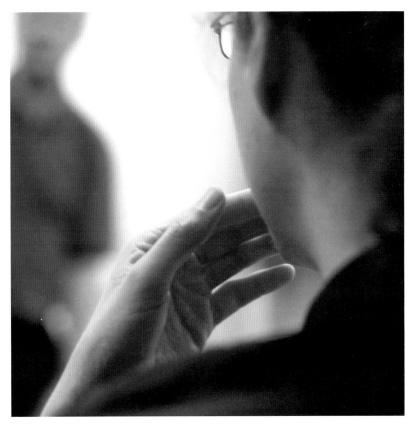

Your GP can give you advice about planning your pregnancy

Understanding your body

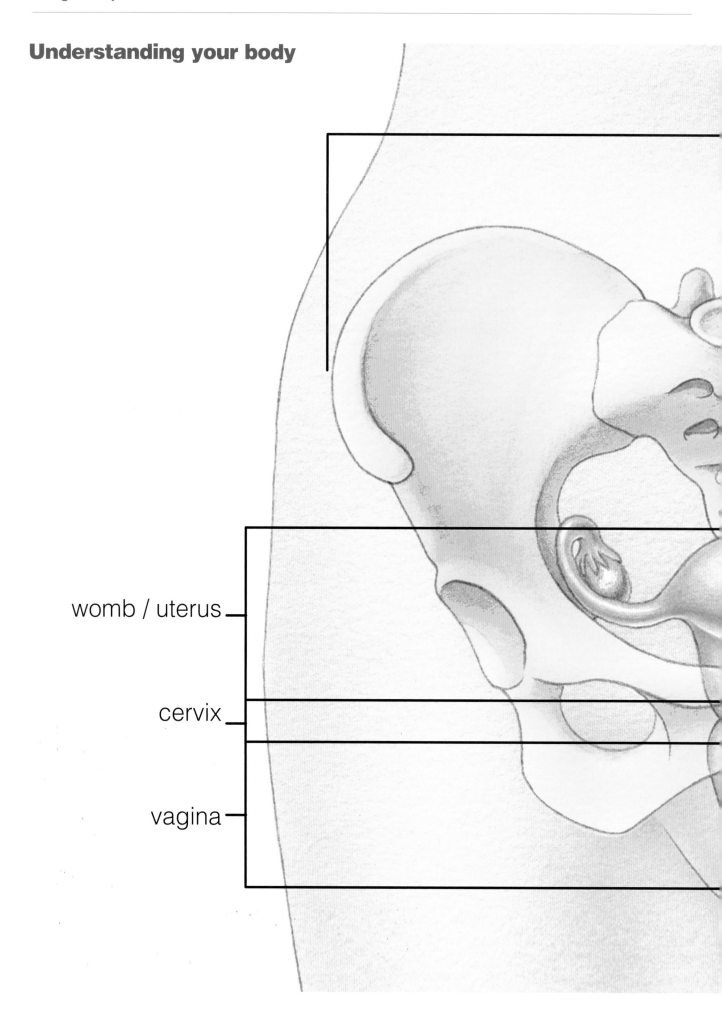

womb / uterus

cervix

vagina

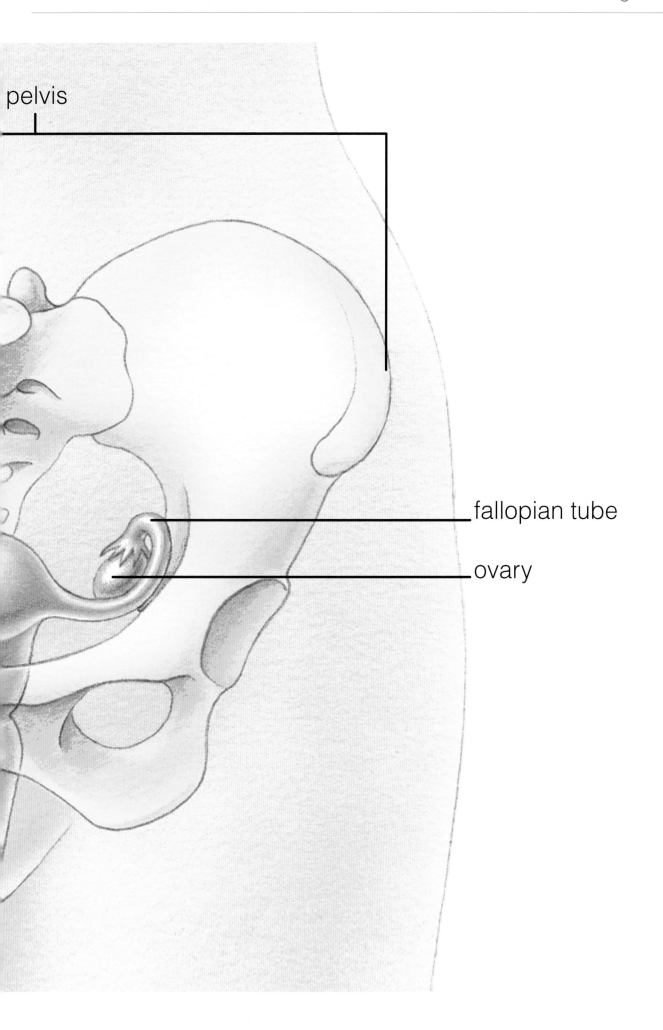

pelvis

fallopian tube

ovary

I have otosclerosis, will it be affected if I get pregnant?

Otosclerosis is a medical condition that causes hearing loss. It may get worse in pregnancy. It is believed that this is because high levels of the hormone oestrogen are released during pregnancy.

If you have otosclerosis and are worried that pregnancy may affect your hearing, get advice from your GP. When you are pregnant it may be necessary to have a hearing test from time to time, to check your hearing. Have a look at RNID's factsheet *Middle ear conditions* for more information.

Can I find out what the chances are of having a deaf baby before I get pregnant?

Yes. All NHS clinical genetic centres can advise deaf and hearing people with a history of deafness in their family, about the chances of having a deaf baby. Your GP can refer you to one of these centres before you get pregnant, but only if you want them to. See RNID's factsheet *Genetics and deafness* for more information.

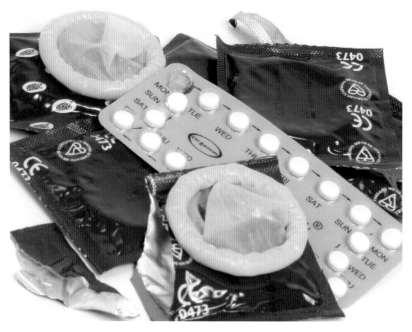

You and your partner will need to stop using condoms if you want to get pregnant

Stop using contraception (birth control)

If you want to get pregnant you will need to stop using contraception. Contraception is something you use to stop getting pregnant.

What sort of contraception do you use?

The pill
You will need to stop taking the pill. Once you have stopped taking it you will need about two months or more to get your periods back to normal. Some women become pregnant quickly after they stop taking the pill, but other women take longer – it could be up to a year or more.

Condoms
There are two types of condom, one for men and one for women. You and your partner will need to stop using condoms if you want to get pregnant.

Contraceptive injections
If you use a contraceptive injection such as Depo-Provera, tell your GP that you want to get pregnant because it could take about six months, or more, after your last injection for you to get pregnant.

Coil/I.U.D
The coil or I.U.D sits in the womb and is usually fitted by your doctor. If you have had one fitted you will need to arrange for your doctor to remove it if you want to get pregnant.

What should I be doing myself while trying for a baby?

There are a few things you can do, even before you get pregnant, to make sure your baby gets the best start in life:

- Eat healthy food and have a balanced diet. It is important for you and the baby. It is also important for your partner to eat healthily. Ask your GP for advice.

- Start taking folic acid. We tell you more about this later in this chapter.

- Talk to your GP about your weight. You may need to put on some weight if you are underweight, or lose some weight if you weigh too much, as this can cause problems during pregnancy. Do not go on a diet unless your GP tells you to. See *Chapter 6 Now you are pregnant – looking after yourself and your baby.*

- Follow an exercise plan. It is a good idea to get fit by exercising *before* becoming pregnant as it helps your body to cope when you do become pregnant. Your GP can advise you if you are not sure where to start.

- Stop drinking alcohol. Drinking can harm your baby. We tell you more in *Chapter 6 Now you are pregnant – looking after yourself and your baby.* It is also good for your partner to cut down on alcohol.

- Stop smoking. Smoking can harm your baby. We tell you more in *Chapter 6 Now you are pregnant – looking after yourself and your baby.* Again, it is good for your partner to cut down on smoking.

- Stop taking illegal drugs. They may harm your baby. If you are taking illegal drugs contact your GP or local drugs service for help and advice on how to stop. We tell you more about this in *Chapter 6 Now you are pregnant – looking after yourself and your baby.* If your partner is taking drugs they should also get help and advice.

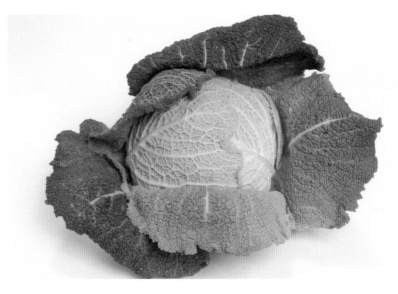

Eat healthy food and have a balanced diet

Taking folic acid when you are trying for a baby

You should take folic acid when you are trying for a baby. Ask your GP about the correct amount to take.

What is folic acid?
Folic acid is part of the B group of vitamins.

Why should I take folic acid?
If you take folic acid it will *help* to prevent your baby developing some serious medical conditions, one of these is spina bifida. However, even if you take folic acid, there may still be a chance that your baby is born with spina bifida.

Women who are pregnant should also take folic acid up to week 13 of their pregnancy. If you don't take it you may also increase your chances of having a miscarriage. From week 13 onwards you have a choice to stop taking folic acid. If you wish to carry on taking it throughout your pregnancy it won't harm you or your baby.

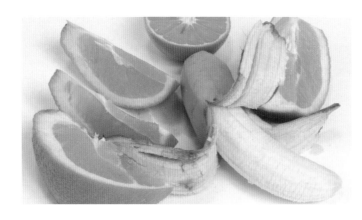

Why do I need folic acid?

You need to take folic acid because it is hard to eat enough foods that are naturally rich in folic acid. As well as taking folic acid, try to eat more food that contains folic acid, for example:

- Leafy green vegetables, for example, brussels sprouts. You should try and eat vegetables lightly steamed, microwaved, or raw.
- Jacket potatoes.
- Black eyed beans.
- Asparagus.
- Wheat germ.
- Bran flakes.
- Papaya.
- Broccoli.
- Oranges.
- Hard-boiled eggs.
- Salmon.

Trouble getting pregnant

If you are having trouble getting pregnant, speak to your GP who will be able to give you advice. They will also be able to refer you for further help if you need it.

Unplanned pregnancy

If you get pregnant and you are not sure what you want to do about it, you might find it useful to speak to your GP or your Family Planning Clinic. They can tell you about the different options available to you.

You might also want to contact an organisation such as Marie Stopes International. They can advise on pregnancy, including unwanted pregnancy and your choices.

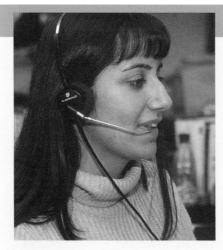

Further information

- www.babycentre.co.uk
- Foresight
- Human Fertilisation and Embryology Authority
- Marie Stopes International
- National Childbirth Trust

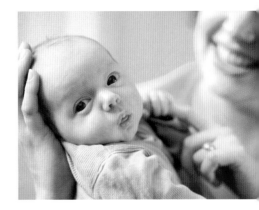

Chapter 3
Finding out you are pregnant

Am I pregnant?

A missed period is one of the first signs that you may be pregnant. There are also other signs to look out for:

- Your breasts might feel tender and a bit bigger than normal.
- You might feel sick.
- You may need to wee more often than usual.
- You may feel very tired.
- You may find you notice smells lots more than normal.
- You may have a metal taste in your mouth.

Pregnancy test

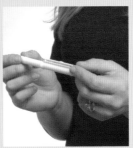

If you think you might be pregnant, you can buy a pregnancy test at a pharmacy (chemist) or you can ask your GP to do a pregnancy test. The test is easy to use and involves testing your urine (wee).

Getting help and information

If you think you are pregnant you should visit your GP or see someone at the health centre as soon as possible. Here are some of the things you might want to ask:

- When will the baby be born?
- Where can I give birth?

- What about my own health?
- What tests are available and should I have them?
- Is there anything in particular I should be eating, or not eating?
- How can I make sure I look after myself and my baby?
- What can I do to help with morning sickness?

Your GP or midwife can also give you a form to fill in, so you can claim free prescriptions and dental treatment for yourself until your baby is one year old.

Working out when your baby will be born

Your GP or midwife will be able to estimate when your baby will be born. This is usually done by adding nine months and seven days to the date when your last period started.
For example:

- The first day of your last period = 12 December.
- Add nine months = September.
- Add seven days = 19.
- Your baby is estimated to be born on 19 September. Remember, this is always an **estimated** date, it does not mean your baby will definitely be born on that date.

Katie's story

Having Deaf parents myself meant I was positive about bringing up my own child. I was excited and wondered how the child would accommodate having a Deaf mother and hearing father. It is still early days as our child is only seven months old.

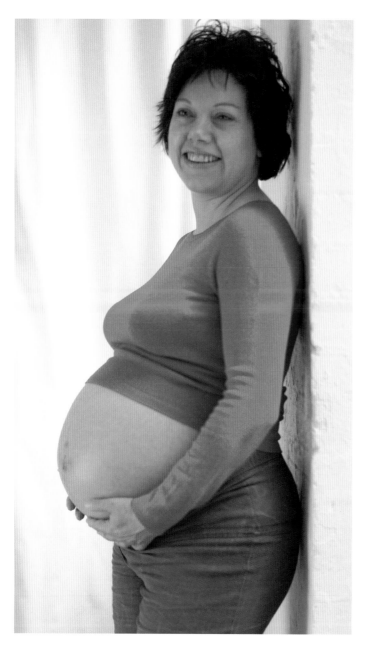

Most babies are born between 37 to 42 weeks after the first day of a woman's last period.

You will also be offered an ultrasound scan which will help work out when your baby is due. See *Chapter 7 Antenatal care* for more information.

Sofia's story

Because my first language is BSL, I really wish all information on pregnancy and birth was available in BSL, but nothing is available. It was difficult to access information from any bookshop or library in general parenting books because of the high level of English and I had to rely on my husband, or someone, to explain the information from English into BSL.

What happens next?

Ask your GP when, and where, you are likely to have appointments with the midwife. In most areas you will be offered a scan when you are around 12 weeks pregnant (see *Chapter 7 Antenatal care*). You may see the midwife before this scan. Women are often surprised at how many appointments they have. Ask who to contact, and how to contact them, if you are concerned about your pregnancy in between appointments.

Your midwife will discuss with you who will look after you during your pregnancy. This depends on where you live. Most care will be provided by a midwife who will visit you at home, or you can visit them at the health centre or GP surgery. You may be offered 'team midwifery' or a 'domino scheme'.

- **Team midwifery**
  A group of midwives will look after you during your pregnancy and after your baby is born. Often, one of these midwives will be with you when you are in labour, whether you have your baby at home or in hospital.

- **Domino scheme**
  Community midwives care for you and one of them will be with you when you have your baby in hospital.

High risk

If you are considered to be a 'high risk' patient, or your pregnancy is 'high risk', you will have more care from the consultant at the hospital. You will also always have a midwife as part of your care.

Paying for an independent midwife

You may want to be looked after by an independent midwife. You have to pay for this option. Ask your GP, or contact the Independent Midwives Association for information.

Your feelings about being pregnant

Everybody reacts differently to the news that they are going to be having a baby. There is no 'right' way to feel once you find out.

Communication support

You will probably also want to ask your GP or midwife to arrange a BSL/English interpreter or other kind of communication support:

- For the 'booking visit' – your first meeting with the midwife.
- For the rest of your pregnancy.
- For parent education classes, these are also called antenatal classes, or parenting classes.
- During the labour and birth.
- After your baby is born, for example, when you are in hospital or when the midwife or health visitor visits you and your baby.

If your first or preferred language is BSL and you find it hard to follow the pregnancy information which your GP, health centre, or midwife gives you, you could ask:

- For an appointment to go through the information.
- To have the information explained to you in BSL.
- To have it written in plain English.
- To be given the information in signed and subtitled videos.

Your GP or midwife may not be very deaf aware – you could suggest they contact a deaf organisation such as RNID or British Deaf Association for more information. See *Chapter 19 Your rights under the Disability Discrimination Act (1995)* for more information.

Patricia's story

When I announced my pregnancy to my family, it was funny and so special! We were at the dinner table, all my family were all together specially for my brother to announce his engagement, I chipped in afterwards and told them I had a surprise for them and announced my pregnancy! It was certainly a special moment, with all the family around us, and clearly they were overjoyed. Especially my dad as I'm the first one in my family to have a child and therefore a first grandchild for my dad.

Bella's story

When I found out I was pregnant I was so shocked as it was unplanned. A few days later, I went to see a doctor. An interpreter was present and the doctor referred me to a midwife. I told the midwife I needed to have an interpreter throughout my pregnancy and I wanted to choose the interpreter who is also my friend. Later on, [in the pregnancy] my GP was trying to make me choose other ways to have someone who can relay for me, for example, asking if my partner is hearing (actually Colin is Deaf), or a hearing friend or my mum, because the interpreting fees are high and they wanted to save money. I was determined and explained to the midwife that I preferred having a professional interpreter rather than using my mum or hearing friend.

At 19 weeks pregnancy, I received a fax from the midwife saying she had found a midwife who can sign. I thought, if she signs at Level 1*, then I'd forget it. Both midwives came to my place and I signed without my voice. [The midwife who can sign] understood me, though not that brilliantly, just above Level 2*.

From 20 weeks pregnancy, the signing midwife looked after me. Gradually, I got used to her style of BSL and I was happy to have her as my midwife as we understood each other.

I appreciated her being there as a 'communicator' for Colin and me when I was in labour for 25 hours. When I arrived at hospital, I was aware that the midwife couldn't do both jobs as communicator and midwife. The other midwife, who can't sign, was responsible for my birth, while my midwife signed to us what the non-signing midwife said. Fourteen hours at home and 11 hours in hospital – yes the midwife stayed with me throughout the time except an hour lunch. I didn't feel panic as the midwife was always there for me. After 25 hours, Colin and I were so happy to see our daughter coming out at long last!

* BSL Level 1 and BSL Level 2 are qualifications in British Sign Language. They do not include any interpreting skills.

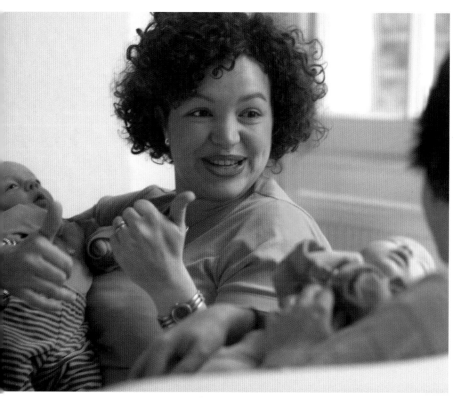

Share your feelings with someone you can trust

Jennifer's story

I have two daughters.

With the eldest, I had my regular community midwife, Sally, who could sign BSL Level 2*. To start off with, I had a midwife who was difficult to understand so I asked for an interpreter for each antenatal appointment. The midwifery manager asked me to try Sally. It was very useful to have her but she wasn't able to sign some words. I was happy to have her just for my antenatal appointments, as these meetings were brief and basic. I had interpreters for my hospital appointments such as having scans or meeting consultants. I was lucky as Sally offered to meet me at my house for appointments so we had time to talk about my pregnancy and preparing for the birth.

Before the birth I wasn't able to book National Childbirth Trust antenatal sessions** as they were fully booked so I attended NHS antenatal sessions with interpreters, but I was disappointed because there were too many of us (about 15 couples).

At the birth, things didn't work out the way I wanted as I was induced, I then had a low dose epidural and my baby was pulled out using a ventouse*** which was a bit traumatic. The most positive thing about this birth was that I had Sally and a good friend who could interpret for me just in case Sally couldn't sign some words or was busy with the delivery. I understood everything throughout the labour

Useful tips

- Share your feelings with your partner or someone you can trust.
- Don't be afraid to ask for support, either from your partner, friends, family or someone you can trust. "My husband was supportive from day one, and that helped me so much."
- If you are worried about anything to do with your pregnancy speak to your GP or midwife.
- Be assertive about your right to communication support, for example, ask for a BSL/English interpreter for your GP or midwife appointments or antenatal classes. See *Chapter 19 Your rights under the Disability Discrimination Act (1995)*.
- Be aware of your own feelings, which can change during the pregnancy. You may feel happy that you are pregnant but if your pregnancy is unplanned you may feel resentful or unhappy. You need to deal with these feelings – speak to your GP, midwife, your partner, or someone you can trust.
- If you are worried about money, find out about benefits you may be able to get. Contact the Maternity Alliance for further information.
- If you need advice and information contact an organisation such as DPPi or National Childbirth Trust. See *Chapter 21 Further information* for details.

and birth, especially when I wasn't sure about having an epidural (as I was afraid of needles) and I was able to ask lots of questions about it to make an informed decision. I think it would have been a lot worse if I hadn't had help with communication.

I was determined to book National Childbirth Trust antenatal sessions with interpreters for my second child. It was so positive and I was well informed this time about birth options and how to help myself throughout my labour. I also learnt that I had the right to change midwifes if I wasn't happy and to choose how I wanted to cope throughout labour.

I had a lovely midwife, Emma, and had antenatal appointments at my home with interpreters at my request. I asked Emma to be on call because I didn't want interpreters at the birth and I was familiar with her way of communicating and vice versa. She organised herself, along with two other midwifes, to be on call for me. At first it was a bit difficult because this is not usually allowed but Emma's manager agreed to let her organise this. As a result of this, I had Emma at the birth of my second baby, that was lovely because she knew what I wanted for the birth and we understood each other. The most important thing was that she had the right attitude.

I had the most fantastic birth. I chose only to have TENS and gas and gave birth when standing up and breastfed her when she was only an hour old. I was able to bond quickly with her. We all went home just four hours after birth, which was great!

*   BSL Level 2 is a qualification in British Sign Language. It does not include any interpreting skills.

** See *Chapter 7 – Antenatal care* for more information.

***See *Chapter 10 – Labour and birth* for more information.

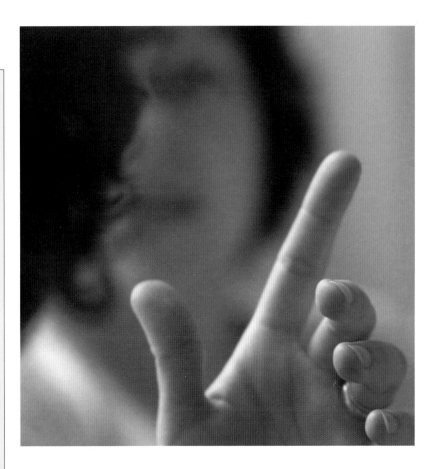

Anja's story

I think that pregnancy gives you the biggest confrontation with being deaf, and deafness as a medical model. You see so many different professionals, so there is the issue of communication, but also everybody asks you about being deaf, why you are deaf, and even how you are going to look after the baby. And when the baby is born, the first thing they will ask about is whether the baby is deaf. It is really something you need to be prepared for. I've found it degrading and humiliating. But luckily there have been nice people too, who weren't bothered about it, and the baby is not interested in it at all!

Sofia's story

After a few years of trying for another baby it came as a great surprise when I got pregnant by assisted conception – IVF*. Because my last pregnancy ended in miscarriage, my husband and I decided not to announce it to our family and friends until passing the 20 weeks into pregnancy, for fear of miscarriage. When five months passed – I was enjoying the pregnancy and my bump was getting bigger, so we decided to announce it only to our close family and friends.

*In Vitro Fertilisation.

What to buy for your baby and your home

Now that you're pregnant you'll probably want to start buying things for your baby. It is also a good time to start making your home safe for your baby. You can buy things like baby monitors but there are also lots of things you can do that don't cost a lot of money, for example, making sure you can't slip on any rugs you might have and putting emergency contact numbers up where you can easily find them. Visit www.parentcentre.co.uk or contact the National Childbirth Trust for more information about making your home safe.

Ask other parents

If you're not sure what to buy for your baby it's a good idea to ask other parents with newborn babies – it might give you an idea where to start. Ask them if they can give you second hand clothing or equipment. *But don't use second hand mattresses or car seats – they will not be so safe.*

Something for your baby to sleep in

You could choose a crib, Moses basket or carrycot. You will need:
- Several cotton sheets.
- Several cotton cellular blankets.
- A **new**, firm, mattress that fits in the cot well.

You might also like to buy:
- A baby monitor.
- A room thermometer.
- An autofade nightlight.

Rosie and Sam's story

Rosie

My period was late – I put that down to stress because at that time, I was very busy with work – so I did the pregnancy test myself and it came out positive. I couldn't believe it. I thought I wouldn't get pregnant but then I was pregnant. I was shocked.

That day, I remember, my partner was off work and at the same time, we were preparing for our wedding. When I showed him the pregnancy test and told him that I was pregnant he was gobsmacked.

Sam

When Rosie gave me the pregnancy test I looked at it and then I looked at her, shocked and unable to say anything . . . it was like every word we said was 'aaaaa' – no other words came out. We were shocked and speechless . . . we just couldn't believe it. But at the same time, we just laughed, felt awkward, felt funny, felt like crying and kept thinking . . . what . . . what . . . what do we do next?

Rosie

It was like a joke, as if it was not really happening, but it was – I was really pregnant!

Sam

It actually took us a long while before we overcame the shock and managed to say a word! It felt like that moment was forever but really it happened in the space of 10 to 15 minutes.

Rosie

We went to see the doctor on the same day to double-check. The doctor said "you're pregnant . . . is that good or bad news?" I smiled and the doctor said "OK, see you in six weeks time" and I was thinking, "six weeks time! But what will happen in the meantime?"

We left and went to a local café for a cup of coffee. It's funny but at that time we just noticed that there were prams and babies everywhere, before we discovered that I was pregnant we never really noticed that sort of thing. So from there on, Sam and I started talking about my pregnancy and quickly, we got used to the idea and went with the flow.

Telling your friends and family about your pregnancy

Many people choose to wait before they tell family and friends they are going to have a baby. Rosie and Sam decided to tell people when Rosie was three months pregnant.

Because our house had been re-decorated we decided to have an open day for our friends and family to pop in to view our house! We invited lots of people and made them welcome to visit us anytime through the day.

On that day, we secretly wore badges. I was wearing an 'I'm going to be a mum' badge and Sam an 'I'm going to be a dad' badge. When we greeted people coming through the front door, we said nothing about the pregnancy. They instantly saw our badges and looked in our eyes to check whether it was true. We smiled and said "yes we're pregnant". So that was a perfect way to announce our pregnancy.

Baby monitors for deaf parents

Lots of parents choose to buy baby monitors so they will know when their baby is crying even if they're not in the same room as them.

How do baby monitors for deaf people work?

Baby monitors for deaf people have two parts:

- A monitor unit, which picks up the sound your baby makes.
- A parents' unit.

The parents' unit has a vibrating pad and it may have a flashing light to attract your attention when you are awake. A vibrating pad will be better at waking you than a flashing light. At night you must use a plug-in vibrating pad to make sure you are woken up.

See your baby on television

You can also get baby monitors that let you see your baby on your television. They have two parts:

- A baby monitor that has a built-in television camera with sound monitoring.
- A parents' unit that plugs into your television.

The built-in television camera on most monitors is sensitive enough to 'see in the dark', so you can see your baby on the television screen even when the room your baby is sleeping in is dimly lit or dark. When your baby cries, the parents' unit connected to your television will automatically interrupt television viewing and switch to the camera monitoring the baby. Most systems also play the sounds your baby makes through the loudspeaker on your television. The picture of your baby on television may not be bright enough to wake you if you are asleep, so you should not rely on this to wake you.

Multi-purpose equipment with a baby monitor

You can also get multi-purpose equipment that alerts you to more than one sound around your home. Modern systems use a pager to alert you to a range of sounds including a baby monitor.

Where can I get a baby monitor for deaf people?

For more information contact:

- **RNID Information Line for our factsheet** *Baby monitors – information for deaf and hard of hearing people.*
- **Visit RNID Sound Advantage at www.rnidshop.com to buy baby monitors**
- **Visit www.rnid.org.uk where you can search RNID's equipment database.**
- **National Deaf Children's Society.**

Julie's story

I was a bit apprehensive about coming home with my new baby and worried how I would cope. The first night was difficult but I managed to get through. My midwife came to visit us at home, checking on our progress and we were doing so well. I have a baby alarm with a vibrating pad which I use at night. This alerting device is invaluable to me because it helps to alert me when the baby cries.

Anja's story

My first babyphone was a disaster. It didn't work properly, and the only advantage was that my baby learnt to sleep quickly through the night, because I wasn't there to attend to him, when he woke up crying. The second babyphone I had was much better. Social services was very helpful, because with my third baby they gave me a different babyphone, so I know which child is crying.

Katie's story

I had a baby monitor with a vibrating pager provided by social services prior to the due date. We already had an audio monitor with a light display. The latter was useful as the pager cannot distinguish between a cry or cough. At night the lights were bright enough to wake me up although my maternal instinct played a part in knowing when the baby was crying.*

*Although flashing lights worked for Katie, RNID recommends that you use a monitor, which also has a vibrating pad to wake you at night.

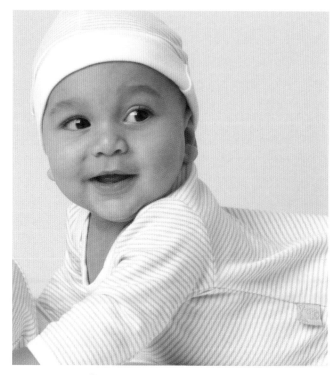

Clothing

To help you choose what clothes your baby will wear remember that most new babies don't like being dressed and undressed, so try and choose clothes that make the job quick and simple. Ask other parents to show you what they used for their babies.

Choose clothes that:
- Are stretchy and have wide neck openings.
- Open at the front.
- Use poppers rather than ties or buttons.
- Open round the top of your baby's legs to make changing nappies easier.
- Are non-flammable – this means they don't catch fire so easily – and don't need ironing.
- Have no rough seams or stitching.

You will need:
- Six to eight sleepsuits/babygros. Buy ones that are suitable for your baby's weight or length, not age. You can get them with built in mittens, which will help stop your baby from scratching herself.
- Two nightgowns. These are easier than sleepsuits to put on and take off quickly and make nappy changing easy at night. Choose ones with a drawstring round the hem so they don't ride up.

- At least four vests or bodysuits but it is a good idea to buy more.
- Two to three pairs of socks.
- Two to three cardigans.
- A light jacket and sunhat to wear in the summer.
- A warm hat, mittens and snowsuit to wear in the winter.

Nappies

You can choose either disposable nappies (you can throw these away) or reusable/washable/cotton nappies.
- **Disposable nappies**
  Buy a few packs – make sure you buy them for newborn babies.
- **Reusable/washable/cotton nappies**
  You can get modern reusable nappies that are specially shaped. You can wash these and use them again. Buy about 24. You'll also need plastic pants, nappy liners, buckets to soak the nappies in and powder to sterilise them.

What are baby clubs?

Most major supermarkets, specialist baby shops and suppliers of baby food and other baby products run their own baby clubs. If you join a club you will be offered free samples, special offers and sometimes a magazine. However, be aware that these are all private companies who will do their best to convince you that their products are the best! If in doubt, ask your health visitor or midwife for impartial advice about what is best for your baby. To find out more about baby clubs, ask at the baby shop or supermarket for information, or look on the packets of baby products.

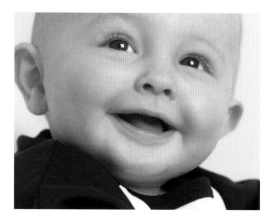

Out and about with your baby

There are lots of different ways you can get around with your baby. Ask other parents, have a look in the shops to see what's available, and use our guide to help you decide:

A baby sling or carrier

These are relatively cheap. You can also use them easily on public transport, in shops, on walks, or off the beaten track. It's a good idea to try various types before you buy to check they are comfortable.

Many baby slings and carriers can be used from birth. Make sure that the baby's head and back are well supported. Backpack style carriers where the baby rides on your back can only be used once your baby can support her head and has a strong back – usually when she can sit upright. There are lots of different carriers and slings so check the instructions.

Don't carry your baby in a sling or carrier after a caesarean section operation (see *Chapter 10 Labour and birth*).

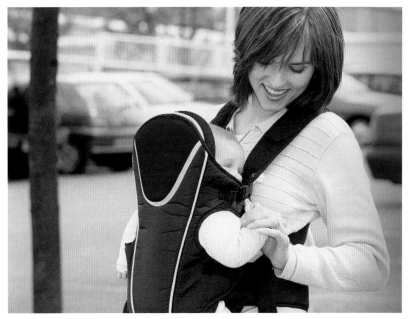
There are lots of different carriers and slings so check the instructions

Tip
If you wear a sling or carrier on your back you can attach a toy with a mirror so you'll be able to see your baby.

A pram or pushchair

A pram or pushchair can be expensive, so find out more before you buy. Do you need one that will fit in your car? Do you want to use it on public transport? Can you fold it easily while holding your baby in your other arm? You can choose between:

- **A traditional pram**
- **A two-in-one or convertible pushchair**
  This can be used flat for a newborn baby, or with an upright back for when your baby has head and neck control.

- **A two-in-one-plus**
  This comes with a seat that can be used for carrying a sleeping baby. However, it is not suitable for your baby to sleep in overnight.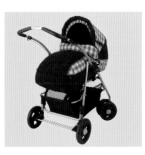
- **A three-in-one or combination pushchair**
  This is like a two-in-one but comes with a lift-off carrycot. If you buy a special mattress, the carrycot can be used for overnight sleeping.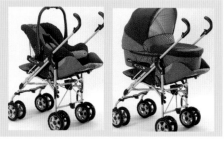
- **A travel system**
  This has everything that a three-in-one or combination pushchair has, plus a car seat that can be locked on to the pushchair.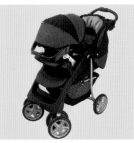
- **An umbrella buggy**
  This is easy to fold up quickly. It is not suitable for a newborn baby or a baby that cannot sit.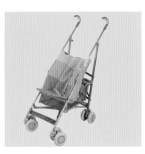

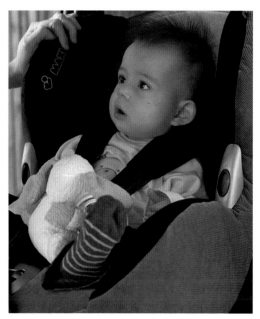

Check that you know how to fit the seat and put a baby in it safely, before you have your baby

Car seats

If you have a car, you will need a car seat suitable for a newborn baby. Most hospitals want you to put your baby in a baby car seat to travel home after the birth because this is the safest way to transport your baby. You can either get a baby seat that can be used until the baby is about nine months old, or a combined baby/child seat.

Using car seats safely

- **Never buy a second hand car seat.**
- Check that you know how to fit the seat and put a baby in it safely, before you have your baby. Your local police station will be able to offer advice. Many offer checks for free. Also check with the shop when you buy the seat.
- Rear-facing seats are safer for small babies. **Never use a car seat in the front passenger seat if your car has air bags.**
- Don't let a baby sleep in a car seat for a long time because the weight of her upper body will mean she can't breathe so well after she has been sleeping upright in a car seat for a while. See if you can buy a car seat that can tip back a bit to help change your baby's position so that she is lying down more.

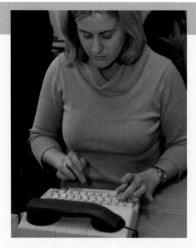

Further information

- The Association for Improvements in the Maternity Services
- www.babycentre.co.uk
- DPPi
- Independent Midwives Association
- Maternity Alliance
- National Childbirth Trust

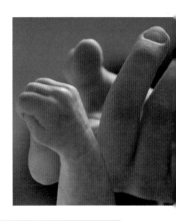

Chapter 4
How your baby grows

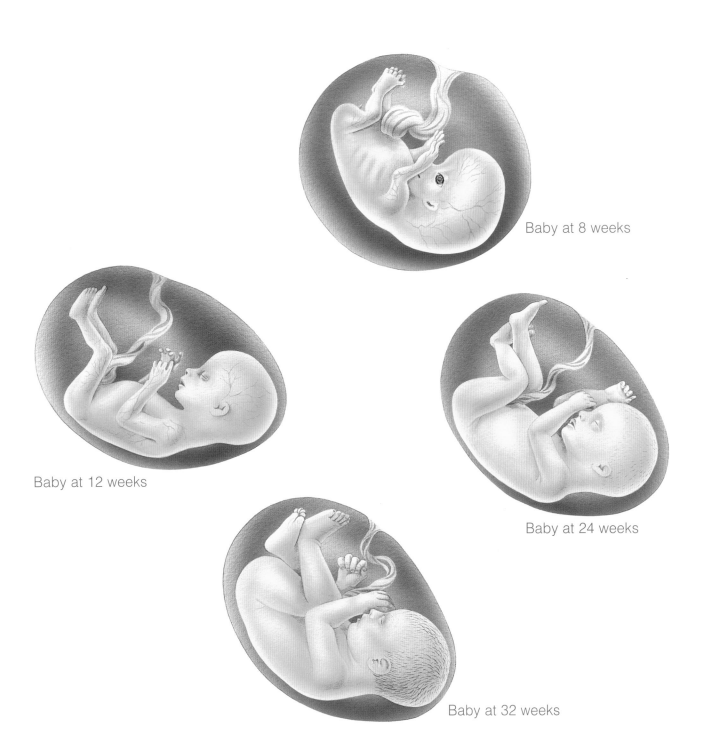

Baby at 8 weeks

Baby at 12 weeks

Baby at 24 weeks

Baby at 32 weeks

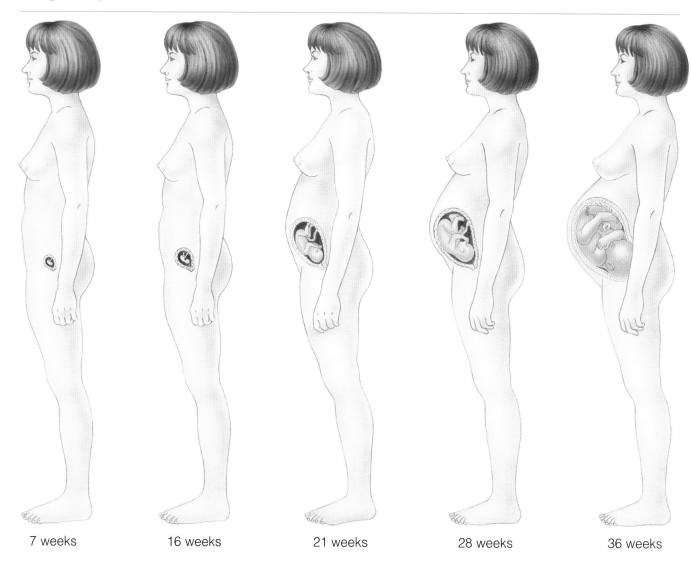

| 7 weeks | 16 weeks | 21 weeks | 28 weeks | 36 weeks |

Your baby at seven weeks

At seven weeks your baby will be a tiny embryo with a heart. She will be about 18mm long. Embryo is the word used to describe a baby up to the beginning of the third month of pregnancy. After three months she's known as a foetus. This is also spelt fetus.

Your baby at two months

Your baby will about 2.5cm long. She will have tiny limb buds.

Your baby at three months

Your baby will be 8cm long. She will have started to swallow and kick but you will not be able to feel the kicks.

Your baby at four months

You may have felt your baby kick by now but this may not happen till later. She will be covered by downy hair called lanugo. She will have tiny fingers and toes.

Your baby at five months

Your baby will be about 20 to 25cm long. Her skin will be covered by a greasy coating called vernix caseosa which is there to protect her.

Your baby at six months

Your baby will have started to practise breathing and will have eyebrows and eyelids.

Your baby at seven months

Your baby will weigh about 1 kg or 2lb. She will be about 35cm long. She will look a lot like a newborn baby.

Your baby at eight months

Your baby will be putting on weight and building up layers of fat. She will have less lanugo (downy hair). She will probably have turned so that her head is ready to come out first when she is born.

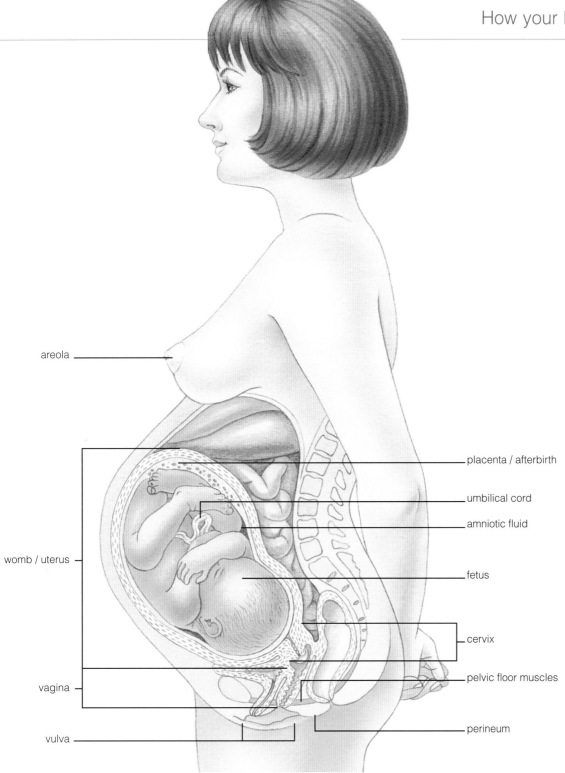

areola

placenta / afterbirth

umbilical cord

amniotic fluid

womb / uterus

fetus

cervix

pelvic floor muscles

vagina

vulva

perineum

Your baby at nine months

Your baby may weigh around 6 to 8lb or 3-4kg and be around 50cm long.

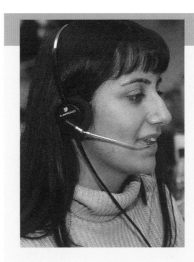

Further information

- www.babycentre.co.uk
- National Childbirth Trust

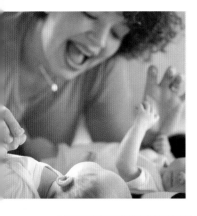

Chapter 5

How your body changes when you are pregnant

As your baby grows you will start to notice changes in your body. Over the next few pages you will find helpful tips to help you cope with some of these changes.

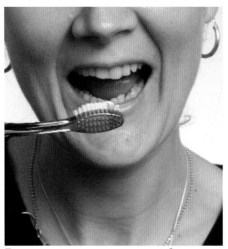

Pregnant women can get free dental treatment on the NHS

Bleeding gums

During pregnancy the gums in your mouth might become soft and spongy. Pregnancy hormones and extra fluid in your body can cause this. Try:

- Gently brushing your teeth with a soft brush, especially near the gums.
- Using dental floss.
- Cutting out sugary food or drinks.
- Remember that pregnant women can get free dental treatment on the NHS, so visit your dentist.

Morning sickness

Does everyone get morning sickness?

Morning sickness is also known as 'pregnancy sickness'. Nearly 80% of women feel sick when they are pregnant. You can feel sick at different times in the day, not only in the morning. You may only feel a little bit sick or you may feel sick every day and may actually vomit. A very few women feel so ill they may need to take time off work. You may start

feeling morning sickness when you are four weeks pregnant. The good news is that most women start to feel a lot better at about 14 weeks into their pregnancy.

What causes morning sickness?

It is believed that hormonal changes during pregnancy may cause morning sickness.

What can I do to help morning sickness?

Eating a snack can help morning sickness. Nibble something at night if you wake up. It may stop you feeling so sick in the morning. Some women have found the following helpful:

- Sucking fresh lemons or peppermints.
- Eating crisps.
- Eating home-made, day-old popcorn.
- Eating crackers.
- Eating ginger biscuits or drinking ginger ale or ginger tea.
- Eating food rich in vitamin B6 such as bananas, breakfast cereals, baked potatoes, lentils and tinned fish.
- Wearing special wristbands that you can buy from the pharmacist.

You should also try to rest as much as you can.

Heartburn

What is heartburn?

Many women get heartburn during pregnancy, especially when the baby gets bigger. It is an unpleasant burning feeling that you usually feel behind your breastbone. You can get the feeling during the day and night. It is often worse when you have eaten, or are lying down. About half of all pregnant women get heartburn and most find it gets better within hours of giving birth.

Heartburn is caused when small amounts of stomach acid leak from the opening at the top of your stomach. The muscle controlling this opening is usually tightly closed, but it becomes looser during pregnancy. As your baby grows it also pushes upwards which can add to the problem.

Constipation

Many women get constipation when they are pregnant, especially near the birth. Constipation means that you cannot go to the toilet (have a poo) so easily. This is because pregnancy hormones soften your muscles so your bowel can't work as well. Sometimes iron supplements can make you constipated. To help:

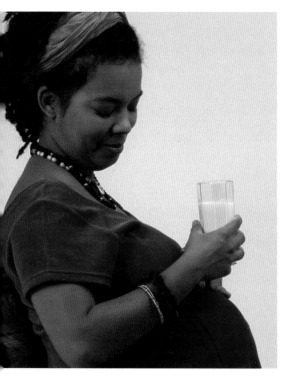

Tips to help with heartburn

- Avoid eating and drinking at the same time.
- Eat six small meals, rather than two or three large ones.
- Avoid eating late at night.
- Avoid fatty and spicy foods.
- Try eating and drinking more dairy products such as plain yoghurt or milk.
- Bend your knees and crouch down to pick things up (instead of bending over).
- Try sleeping propped up on several firm pillows.
- Ask your GP to prescribe an antacid drug.

- Eat more fibre – this is found in fruit and vegetables.
- Drink lots of water – about two litres of water a day.
- Try not to strain (push hard) when you go to the toilet, it may cause piles. Try relaxing and breathing calmly.
- Take more exercise.
- If you feel very uncomfortable you may want to ask your midwife or pharmacist about laxatives, especially near to the date your baby is due to be born (your due date).
- Some complementary medicine may be helpful. If you would like more information about using complementary medicine during pregnancy ask your GP or midwife. You can also contact the National Childbirth Trust, the British Complementary Medicine Association or the Institute for Complementary Medicine (see *Chapter 21 – Further information*).

Tender breasts

When you are first pregnant your breasts may feel tender or tingly. They will also get bigger during pregnancy. This is because your hormones are getting them ready for breastfeeding. Make your breasts more comfortable by:

- Wearing a good support bra to avoid overhang.
- Putting a cold flannel on them if they feel hot.
- Gently massaging them, but take care not to massage too hard.

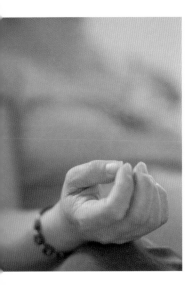

Skin changes

You will notice that your skin changes when you are pregnant, this can happen quite early on:

- It might become more oily or drier than usual.
- Your face may become smoother, but it might also look a bit chubby.
- Quite early on, the skin around your nipples may be darker. You will get a brown line down the centre of your stomach. You may get brown patches on your face too. All these colour changes go away or fade after the baby is born.
- You might get stretch marks on your stomach and your breasts from about three or four months. They will fade after the baby is born but never go away completely.
- You will probably sweat more and feel that your hands and feet are warmer. This is because your body has an increased blood supply and your small blood vessels are expanding (getting wider).

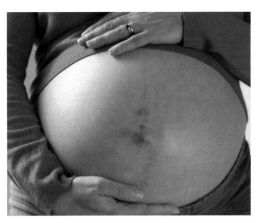

Itching

Some women get itchy skin during pregnancy. It may be all over the body or on your bump. Ask your midwife or GP for advice if:

- The itching is very bad.
- The itching is on the palms or soles of your feet. This may be a sign of a serious condition called 'cholestasis of pregnancy'.
- If you have a rash.
- If you have jaundice.
- If the itching doesn't get better or you feel ill.

If there is no rash it may help to soothe your skin using oils or lotions, cooled water or calamine lotion.

Dizziness

Some women feel dizzy early in pregnancy but it can happen at any time. During pregnancy, you may get low blood pressure. You may find that if you stand for a long time, or get up too quickly this makes you feel dizzy.

- Try not to stand up for long periods of time.
- Get up slowly if you are sitting or lying down.
- Take care when getting out of a hot bath.

If your blood sugar levels are getting too low you may also feel dizzy. It is best to eat small snacks regularly. If you feel faint, sit down and put your head between your knees, loosen any tight clothing and breathe deeply.

Later on in pregnancy you may feel faint if you lie down flat on your back because your womb presses down on you. Try lying on your left side.

Headaches

You may find you get headaches at anytime during your pregnancy. This may be because of hormonal changes, sinusitis, eyestrain or tiredness.

If you get headaches tell your midwife or GP especially if you have high blood pressure (see *Chapter 8 If things go wrong during pregnancy* for information about high blood pressure). Ask your GP or pharmacist for advice about painkillers you can take. **Remember to tell your pharmacist that you are pregnant.**

If you get headaches, try:

- Massaging your scalp with your fingers.
- Cutting out/down on coffee, tea and cola.
- Drinking more water.
- Relaxing and getting plenty of sleep and rest.

Tiredness

You are likely to feel tired if you are pregnant. This is because your body is working very hard to support your developing baby. Your hormones can also make you feel relaxed and sleepy.

It is important to rest as much as possible. Sit down, or lie down, preferably on your left side, as much as you can and try to stretch out with your feet higher than your hips.

Weight change

Some women put on lots of weight when they are pregnant and some woman hardly put on any. It will depend on your own body and what it needs. But check with your midwife if you are concerned about your weight or have bloating.

Don't try to slim
- Aim to eat lots of different types of food and try to make sure you eat a lot of fresh food.
- Add extra portions of bread, cereals, fruit and vegetables to your diet, rather than chocolate, crisps and fizzy drinks.
- If you don't feel like eating much, try to drink healthy drinks instead such as fruit juice and milk-based drinks.

You will find more information about healthy eating in *Chapter 6 Now you are pregnant - looking after yourself and your baby.*

Backache

When you're pregnant the weight of your womb pulls your lower spine forward, putting a strain on your lower back. At the same time pregnancy hormones soften your ligaments. All this can lead to backache. Changes in the way you stand and move may also lead to backache and may also activate an old injury.

Sometimes doing the same movements at work, again and again, can cause backache.

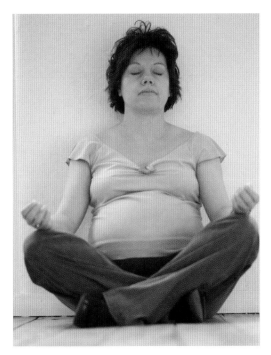

If you get headaches, try relaxing

In the last month of your pregnancy you may get backache because your baby has moved down in your womb and her back is lying against your back. If that happens, try kneeling on all fours from time to time.

Tips to avoid backache

- Do not lift heavy objects. If you have to lift something heavy always bend from your knees, not from your waist, and try not to twist.
- Stand as upright as possible.
- Relax your shoulders.
- Make sure that you stand evenly on both feet.
- Sit against the back of a chair or put a cushion in the small of your back when you are sitting down.
- Try and exercise. Walking and swimming will help keep your back flexible. **However, avoid crawl, butterfly or breaststroke when you are pregnant, or soon after you have had a baby, as pregnancy hormones make your ligaments more stretchy and you could damage joints in your knees or pelvis.** You can do doggy paddle, crawl kick or try floating on your back and using gentle arm movements. Find out about swimming classes for pregnant women.
- Wear a maternity girdle if your backache is really bad.
- Wear flat shoes.
- If you are lying down, turn on your side before trying to get up, and use your arms for support.

Varicose veins

Some pregnant women develop varicose veins, usually later in pregnancy. These can be veins in your leg that become bigger. They can ache and make your legs feel tired or heavy. They do not bother some women, but others find them painful and uncomfortable. A few women develop varicose veins in the vulva and vagina, which can be very painful.

Pregnancy hormones that relax the muscular walls in your veins cause varicose veins. At the same time there is more blood in your body. This makes it more difficult for the muscle in your veins to pump blood around your body. This means that some blood collects lower down in your body. Also, as your womb gets bigger it puts extra pressure on veins in your leg and pelvis area.

You can help prevent varicose veins by:

- Walking and swimming more (see the earlier section on *Tips to avoid backache* for information about swimming safely when you are pregnant).
- Doing special exercises with your feet and ankles, ask your midwife or GP to show you.
- Doing pelvic floor exercises, ask your midwife or GP to show you.
- Never sitting with your knees crossed, or thighs pressing against the edge of a chair.
- Keeping your legs raised when you are sitting.
- Trying not to stand for long periods of time.
- Eating foods rich in vitamin E and vitamin C.

If you already have varicose veins, try:
- All the tips above.
- Wear support tights right from the start of your pregnancy
- Raise the foot of your bed to help the blood drain back to the heart.

Cramp

Some women suffer from cramps in their calves (back of the legs) or feet, in the night.
- It may help if you stretch your feet or legs before bed and sleep with your feet out from under the covers.
- If you do get cramp, massage and flex your foot.

Nosebleeds, stuffy nose or runny nose

You may get nosebleeds at any time during your pregnancy. Pregnancy hormones and extra blood in your body can cause this.
- If you get a blocked nose, try inhaling steam. Ask your GP before taking any medicine or using essential oils to help clear your nose.
- If you get a nosebleed, pinch the end of your nose gently and lean forward slightly. If it does not stop call your GP.
- Also, tell your GP or midwife about your nosebleeds so they can check your blood pressure.

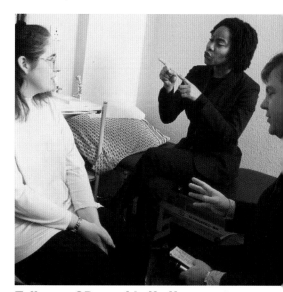

Tell your GP or midwife if you get nosebleeds

Discharge (vaginal discharge)

It is normal to have an increased clear discharge from your vagina when you are pregnant.

Thrush

You may get thrush when you are pregnant. Thrush is a thick, itchy white discharge from your vagina. It is also called a yeast infection. A change in the balance of acids and alkalis in your vagina can cause it. If you get thrush, get advice from your GP. You can try:

- A cream or pessary for thrush. A pessary is medicine that you put in your vagina. **If you buy this over-the-counter, tell the pharmacist you're pregnant.**
- Eating less sugar and more 'live' yoghurt. Have a look on the side of the yoghurt pot to see if it is 'live'.
- Wearing cotton knickers. Don't wear tights or tight trousers.

If you have any other smelly, itchy or coloured discharge get advice from your GP. It could be caused by an infection.

Mood swings

You may find your mood swings from feeling anxious or weepy to feeling well and happy. If you feel very unhappy or can't sleep properly do talk to your midwife and family about any worries that you have.

Bad dreams

You may find you have bad or very vivid dreams when you are pregnant. It may help to tell a sympathetic listener about them. You may find that other women have had similar dreams, which can be reassuring.

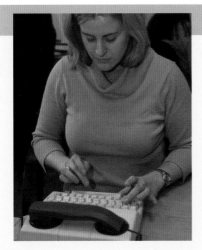

Further information

- National Childbirth Trust

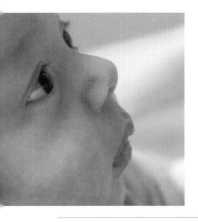

Chapter 6
Now you are pregnant – looking after yourself and your baby

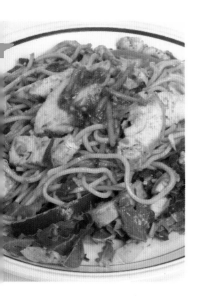

Eat healthily

- Now that you are pregnant your baby is growing inside you. She will need food from you so it is important that you eat well.
- If you have morning sickness and it makes it really hard for you to eat, tell your midwife.
- It's also important to drink plenty of water and other drinks (but not alcohol) to keep your body in good shape and to stop you getting dehydrated (being dry). Try and aim to drink about two litres of water, or more, a day.

Try to get enough protein

- You should try to eat two to three servings a day of lean meat (meat that doesn't have a lot of fat), fish, beans, nuts, or food made from milk, such as cheese.
- Eating pulses and grains together means you will get more protein. Pulses include, for example, beans or chickpeas. Grains include, for example, toast or rice. For example, you could try beans on toast or chickpeas with rice.
- Stir-fry fresh vegetables with chicken, and rice or noodles.
- If you are vegetarian get advice from one of the organisations listed at the end of this chapter.

What should I eat?

Here are some tips to help you follow a healthy diet when you are planning a baby and once you are pregnant.

Eat lots of fresh vegetables and fruit

Vegetables and fruit are full of vitamins and minerals, especially if you eat them raw or lightly cooked.

Snack on starchy carbohydrates

This will also help you if you feel sick. Try:
- Day-old, home-made popcorn.
- Crackers.
- Dry toast.
- Plain boiled rice or pasta.

Aim for an average of six servings of starchy carbohydrates throughout the day. One serving equals:
- Two slices of bread or
- Two chapattis or
- A bowl of breakfast cereal or
- Six tablespoons of boiled pasta or
- Four tablespoons of rice or
- Two potatoes or yams.

Take folic acid

It is important that you take folic acid early in your pregnancy. Get advice from your GP or midwife and see *Chapter 2 Planning a baby* for more information.

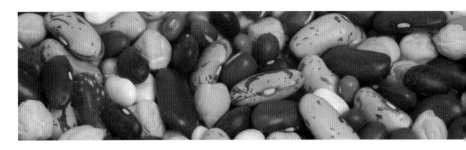

Are there any foods I should stop eating?

It is important that you stop eating certain food when you are pregnant. Eating some foods can lead to health problems which means you could lose or damage your baby.

Listeria

Listeria are bacteria which can cause miscarriage or premature birth. They can also give your baby an infection which could cause pneumonia or meningitis after she has been born.

Foods to avoid

Do **not** eat:

- Soft cheeses, made from unpasteurised milk, such as Brie and Camembert (but it is OK to eat cottage cheese and curd cheese).
- Blue-veined cheeses such as Danish Blue or Stilton.
- Unpasteurised goat's, cow's or sheep's milk. Look on the label and ask for advice if you are not sure.
- Any kind of pâté.
- Uncooked, or under-cooked, ready meals.

Toxoplasmosis

Toxoplasmosis is caused by a parasite in cat and dog faeces (poo), and also in raw meat. It can lead to your baby going blind or getting brain damage.

- Wear gloves when gardening and wash your hands afterwards.
- Try to avoid handling pets or litter trays. If you have to handle pets wear gloves and wash your hands afterwards.
- Wash your hands before handling food.
- Wash all fruit and vegetables before you eat them, even those that you buy washed and packaged already.

- Make sure you cook meat and ready-meals thoroughly.
- Wash kitchen surfaces and your hands after handling meat.

Foods to avoid

Do **not** drink:

- Unpasteurised goat's, cow's or sheep's milk.

Do **not** eat:

- Any kind of pâté.
- Raw or undercooked meat such as Parma ham.

Salmonella

Salmonella is a very unpleasant form of food poisoning.

Foods to avoid

Do **not** eat:

- Raw or soft boiled eggs. You should wash the outside of the egg before boiling it. Boil an egg so that the white and yolk are both firm.
- Food made with raw or soft-boiled eggs, such as mayonnaise, mousse, cake icing, cheesecake, home made ice cream and ready prepared coleslaw. If you make your own coleslaw do not use mayonnaise.
- Chicken and turkey that you have not cooked for long enough. The juices should be clear with no pink colour.
- Raw shellfish, such as crab.
- Smoked and cured meat, and fish, unless you buy it from a shop with a very good reputation, already packed and stamped with a sell-by date.
- Soft-whip ice cream – the sort sold by ice-cream vans.

Remember to wash salad that comes ready prepared in a bag, even if it has already been washed.

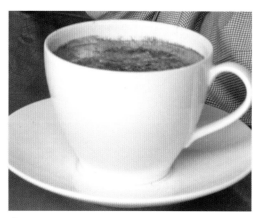

Cut out, or cut down on caffeine

Retinol – one form of vitamin A

If you take too much vitamin A, or if there is too much vitamin A in your food, it can harm your baby.

Foods to avoid
Do **not** eat:
- Liver.
- Any kind of pâté.
- Cod liver oil or any vitamin or mineral supplements containing Vitamin A.

Get advice from your GP or midwife about vitamins or minerals that are safe to take.

Peanut allergies

If you eat peanuts whilst you are pregnant you may increase the chance of your child developing a peanut allergy. You should also avoid eating peanuts if you or any of your family have asthma, eczema, hayfever or a nut allergy.
Foods to avoid
Do **not** eat:
- Peanuts.
- Any foods containing peanuts, for example, peanut butter or satay sauce.

Peanut oil is also called groundnut oil.

Where can I get advice on what to eat?

- Speak to your GP or midwife.
- Contact the organisations listed at the end of this chapter for advice on what to eat during pregnancy and while breastfeeding.

What about coffee, alcohol, smoking and drugs?

It is important to look after yourself and your baby when you are pregnant by cutting out, or cutting down:
- Caffeine.
- Alcohol.
- Tobacco (smoking).
- Illegal drugs.

Caffeine
Caffeine is found in coffee, tea, cola and energy drinks. If you drink too much coffee when you are pregnant you may be increasing your risk of having a miscarriage or your baby being born with a disability. Caffeine might also make your baby grow more slowly during pregnancy.

In a day try not to drink more than:
- Four to five cups of instant coffee or
- Two to three cups of filtered coffee or
- Five to six cups of tea.

Avoid soft drinks that contain cola. Check on the tin.

Tobacco (smoking)
It is very important that you do not smoke when you are pregnant. Tobacco can:
- Slow down your baby's growth.
- Increase the risk of going into labour early.
- Make your baby's heart beat too fast.
- Increase the risk of your baby having a cot death. (See Chapter 14 Your baby's first few weeks at home).

Help with giving up smoking

You can get help to give up smoking. Your midwife can tell you what help is available locally. You can also contact helplines such as Quit or the NHS Pregnancy Smoking Helpline for extra support.

Alcohol
Drinking alcohol can harm your baby. Some women choose not to drink at all for the first three months of their pregnancy. Many women 'go off' alcohol during pregnancy but some women don't. It is

sensible not to drink any more than one or two units of alcohol once or twice a week. One unit of alcohol is, for example:

- Half a pint of ordinary strength beer, lager, or cider.
- One small glass of wine.
- One single measure of spirits.

You may have been drinking without realising you were pregnant. If you are worried, it may help to talk to your GP or midwife.

Help with giving up alcohol

If you need help and support to cut down the amount of alcohol you drink talk to your GP, or midwife. You can also contact Alcohol Concern.

Illegal drugs

Illegal drugs include, for example, cannabis, cocaine, heroin, acid (LSD) and ecstasy.

If you are taking illegal drugs:

- Ask your GP or midwife for advice and information about how they will affect your baby and for help in giving them up.
- Contact your local drugs service. You will find them listed in your Yellow Pages telephone directory.

Over-the-counter drugs

You should stop taking some drugs you can buy over-the-counter at the pharmacy, these include painkillers, cough medicines and cold cures. Ask your pharmacist, GP or midwife for advice before taking them and remember to tell your pharmacist you are pregnant before you buy any drugs.

Sex during pregnancy

It is safe for you and your baby if you have sex when you are pregnant, unless your doctor or midwife tells you not to. You may find you enjoy sex even more, or you might go right off it. However you feel about sex, don't worry about it. If you do have concerns, try and share them with your partner and get advice from your GP or midwife.

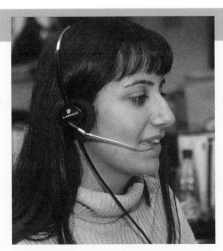

Further information

- Alcohol Concern
- Drinkline
- Eating for pregnancy helpline
- National Childbirth Trust
- NHS Pregnancy Smoking Helpline
- Quit

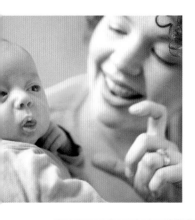

Chapter 7
Antenatal care

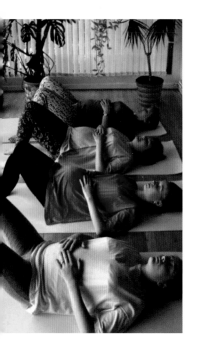

Antenatal care means the care you and your baby are given before your baby is born.
Ante = before. Natal = birth.

As well as getting care from medical professionals, remember that your friends and family can also be a great source of support.

Sofia's story

I got closer to my sister-in-law and her experience of pregnancy really helped me to understand what was happening with my own pregnancy, I felt I could ask her anything and she was so supportive. As a regular to Deaf community events, I have had lots of support from my Deaf friends especially with advice about food and drinks – what is good and not good for pregnancy – which I found useful.

Anna's story

I had poor access to communication support during antenatal classes. I had a 'communicator' but she was Level 1*. The hospital booked her. I missed out on lots of information. I saw a video about preparing for labour but it had no subtitles and no BSL translation on the video. The communicator wasn't much help as I didn't understand the video.

I would have preferred to go to antenatal classes specifically for deaf parents so that I was in a signing environment. Maybe I would have understood more from those classes and shared more enthusiasm with other deaf parents. Instead, I had classes where I was the only Deaf parent and I was so isolated, I couldn't interact with other parents so I become quiet and felt left out from the chit-chats between them.

*BSL Level 1 is a qualification in British Sign Language. It does not include any interpreting skills.

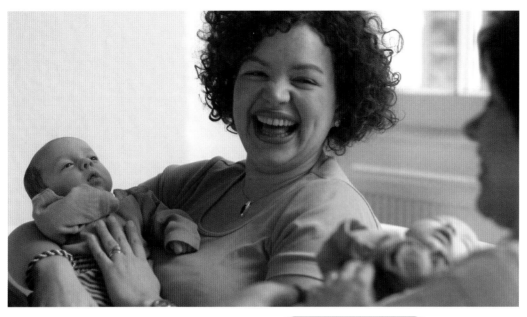

NHS antenatal classes

Ask your GP or midwife about antenatal classes. The NHS usually provides these free of charge. They will cover such things as:

- Exercises, such as pelvic floor exercises.
- Preparing for the birth.
- What labour is like.
- Pain relief in labour.
- Having a caesarean birth. We tell you more about this in *Chapter 10 Labour and birth*.
- Looking after yourself after the birth.
- Being a new mum.
- The local maternity unit, where you might have your baby.

National Childbirth Trust antenatal classes

You can also go to National Childbirth Trust antenatal classes – these are held all over the UK. You will have to pay for these but the National Childbirth Trust will be able to help you if you can't afford to pay. The classes offer support and give you the chance to make friends, share worries and concerns, compare how you feel and get information to help you make the best choices for you. Your partner will also be able to get involved. To find out more contact the National Childbirth Trust.

You may find that NHS classes are often larger than National Childbirth Trust ones.

Rosie's story

I found lots of barriers accessing information and services. For example, when Sam, my husband, and I had to go to antenatal classes, no interpreter was booked. I was told to find one and when I found one, I was told to pay for the interpreter services. Why should I? I had to fight with the Health Authority to pay and ended up using my Access to Work fund to pay for it.* It's wrong. It should have been the Heath Authority's responsibility to pay for the interpreter under the Disability Discrimination Act. So I had to miss the first antenatal class to find an interpreter and booked her for the rest of the classes. Also, I later found out that the Health Authority do, in fact, have a contract with RNID interpreting services but many of the health professionals are not aware of this.**

*Access to Work is a government-funded programme that supports deaf and disabled people who are in work or looking for work. It provides advice and information and can help pay for equipment and communication support in the workplace.

** See *Chapter 20 Information for health professionals*.

Michael's story

When we wanted to attend the local health centre's antenatal classes, we made some enquiries to see whether they would provide a sign language interpreter. I was amazed that they would not provide interpreting support for a deaf father if his partner is not deaf. Fortunately, we were able to push the matter further. Due to our demands, they finally provided sign language support throughout the classes.

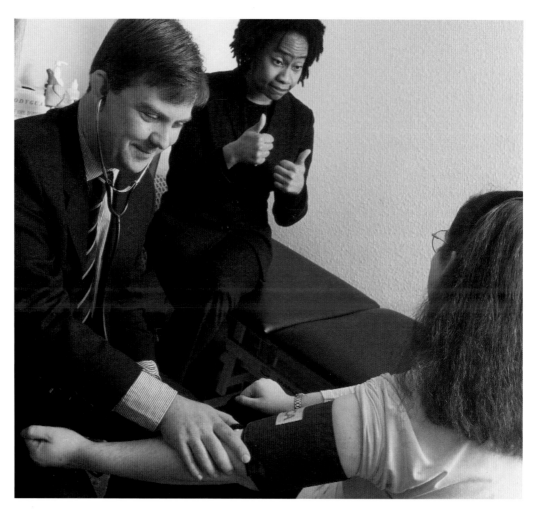

Rosie's story

My mum is so good with me – she explained how her pregnancy went when she had me. My friends are also a great support, but it depends on whether they have children of their own. If they have children, it's great talking to them about issues around kids and sharing experiences on child development, how to deal with a baby crying, breastfeeding and what all mothers are going through!

Patricia's story

I have friends who have children of their own that I can turn to for emotional and peer support. I've learned so much from my friends, especially those who are expecting a baby or have children, and we share experiences on raising our own babies and children. I have also learned from reading suitable books on parenting.

What sort of antenatal care will I get?

Your midwife will see you regularly when you are pregnant to check that all is well with you and your baby.

The **booking visit** is the name of the first meeting you have with the midwife or GP. They will ask you for lots of information and you can ask them lots of questions. Your antenatal care will also be planned during this visit. It's a good idea to talk about communication support at this visit.

The midwife will usually see you at your GP surgery, health centre, maternity unit or at home:
➡ Every four weeks – until you are 28 or 30 weeks pregnant.
➡ Then every two weeks – until you are 36 weeks pregnant and
➡ Then every week after that.
But this depends on where you live. In some parts of the country you will be seen less often.

Farah's story

Booking a sign language interpreter with the midwife was difficult because she did not know how to book the interpreter. Even though I explained that there was a poster outside about it she said she didn't know. Also, the poster I saw outside was for different spoken languages. I noticed that BSL was not included in the list, does that mean deaf people are not entitled to have access to interpreting services?

I saw a different midwife each time, the first one was unhelpful, especially with booking an interpreter, but the second midwife had a positive attitude – she doesn't sign but said she had a deaf relative and that helps.

Often, I went to see the midwife with my mum, but what annoyed me the most is that the midwife talked to my mum about my condition, not me. Why can't they talk to me directly? I may be Deaf but I'm not stupid, I need to know what is happening – it's my pregnancy, not my mum's.

Also, it is clear on my maternity record that I am Deaf and need a BSL interpreter, they used a 'hearing scheme' label* on my appointment card and on my file, but the staff were still not deaf aware. They still called out my name without getting my attention! Every single time, the same thing happens.

However, on a positive note, when I went to hospital, I found one particular midwife so helpful. We had clear communication by fax. She was naturally concerned when I missed my appointment for a check-up. It's rare to see someone so positive.

*Hearing Concern publish ear symbol stickers which medical professionals can stick onto patient's records (contact details in *Chapter 21 Further information*).

What sort of tests will I be offered?

You will be offered a range of antenatal tests and checks but it is up to you to decide if you want them done.

Your midwife or GP will offer to:
- Check your blood pressure – at every antenatal visit.
- Check your weight and height – usually only at your first meeting, unless you have very clearly lost or gained weight.
- Examine your heart and lungs – usually only at the first visit.
- Test your urine (wee) to check your sugar levels, and for any infections – at every visit.
- Feel your abdomen to see the size of your womb – at every visit.
- Ask about your general health – at every visit. Tell them if you are worried about anything, for example, any unusual discharge from your vagina.
- Check if you have swollen hands, ankles or feet – at every visit.
- They may, very occasionally, ask to do an internal examination. They should explain what they are doing, and why, and get your permission.

It may help you to make a list of things you want to discuss beforehand. You may want to take your partner, or friend, with you who can remind you of any questions you want to ask.

Communication support

- Tell the antenatal tutor in advance that you are deaf and ask them to arrange communication support.
- You may need to tell the tutor how you prefer to communicate in the class. The tutor may not have worked with deaf mothers-to-be before, so you may want to meet beforehand to talk about communication.
- Some antenatal classes may use relaxation techniques that involve turning off the lights or shutting your eyes, so discuss this with the tutor before the class starts.
- If you are having problems getting support in NHS classes, ask to speak to the Midwifery Manager or the Supervisor of Midwives on call.

Will I be offered other tests?

Yes. You will also be offered tests to see if you, or your baby, have specific medical conditions. You will usually have to go to hospital to have these tests although your GP or midwife may carry out some blood tests at your GP surgery or health centre. Before you have the tests try and find out as much as you can about them, so that you know what to expect and what they are for.

There are two sorts of tests:

- A **screening** test tells you what your *chances* are of having a baby with a condition such as Down's syndrome or spina bifida. It does not actually tell you if your baby has one of these conditions. Screening tests are sometimes done by ultrasound scan – which does not involve inserting a needle into your womb or piercing your skin – and sometimes by blood tests.
- A **diagnostic** test can tell for certain whether your baby has a condition such as Down's syndrome or spina bifida. Diagnostic tests involve taking small samples from inside your womb.

Elizabeth's story

I became hard of hearing in my mid-twenties, but actually lost a lot of hearing almost overnight when I got pregnant with my daughter who is now two years old. So, the first couple of months of pregnancy were an ordeal, as I had to cope with my hearing loss and the fact that my pregnancy was unplanned.

I went for my first scan with my husband. I was excited and looking forward to seeing my baby on the scan for the first time. We were in a room with a scan machine. While I was having my first scan, the doctor was talking directly to my husband. I hadn't a clue what was being said and have never felt so isolated and left out.

Also don't forget that I suddenly became deafened quickly during my pregnancy so I didn't get the chance to master the art of lipreading. My hearing aids at the time were so bad that I couldn't hear a word at all due to interfering noises.*

* One solution the staff could have tried would have been to write everything down.

They may involve piercing your skin or your womb with a fine needle. It can hurt when the needle enters the womb and so you may be offered a local anaesthetic to help you feel less pain. These tests have a slight risk of miscarriage.

Blood tests

You will be offered blood tests to:
- Find out your blood group and if you are Rhesus positive or negative and if there are any Rhesus antibodies in your blood.
- Check your iron levels to see if you are anaemic.
- See if you have been vaccinated against rubella (German measles).
- Test for certain infections.
- Find out if you are HIV positive. This is a virus, which can lead to a medical condition called AIDS.

Testing for Down's syndrome

You will also be offered blood tests at about 15-16 weeks to see if you are at risk of having a baby with Down's syndrome or spina bifida. This is a **screening** test. This test looks at the level of hormones in your blood.

- **Screen negative**
  Usually if the test shows that your risk of being pregnant with a baby with Down's syndrome is less than 1 in 250, your result will be described as *screen negative*. This does not mean that you definitely aren't pregnant with a baby who has Down's syndrome – it only means that it is very unlikely.
- **Screen positive**
  If your blood test shows that your risk is more than 1 in 250, your result will be described as *screen positive*. This means that your risk of having a baby with Down's syndrome is higher and you may want to have further tests, such as an amniocentesis, to confirm whether or not your baby has Down's syndrome *(see later for more information)*.

Women over 35 years have a higher risk of having a baby with Down's syndrome.

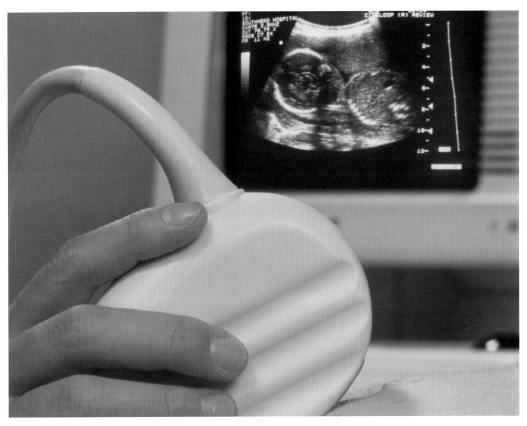

An ultrasound scan allows you to see what your baby looks like when she is lying in your womb

The ultrasound scan

What is an ultrasound scan?

An ultrasound scan allows you to see what your baby looks like when she is lying in your womb. High frequency sound waves are used to build up a picture. You will see this picture on what looks like a television screen. You will need to go to hospital to have an ultrasound scan.

Communication support during your scan

When a scan is done, it is normal for the technician to turn the screen away from you at first so that they can look at it and do all the measurements. This can take some time, and the technician may not communicate with you while they are doing this.

Then they will normally turn the scan towards you and explain what they can see. Sometimes the lighting in the room may be low and it may be difficult for you to lipread. It is particularly important to ask the hospital to arrange communication support or to take

someone with you who can help explain what is going on. You should also ask the technician to explain what happens during the scan before they begin.

Why do I need a scan?

The scan will help you know:
- If you are having more than one baby, for example, twins or triplets.
- Whether your baby is growing and developing properly.
- When your baby will be born as it can show the size of the baby.
- If your baby will be a boy or a girl but it's not always easy to tell.

Sharon's story

Both my two pregnancies were healthy so I did not have any major fears. I read everything I could find and I attended two sets of antenatal classes – one run by the NHS and the other run by the National Childbirth Trust. I found [the National Childbirth Trust course] extremely valuable and informative as it was much more in depth and there were plenty of group discussions – I had an interpreter. Using an interpreter helped improve Deaf awareness, and created interest in learning to sign so I made some very good friends there.

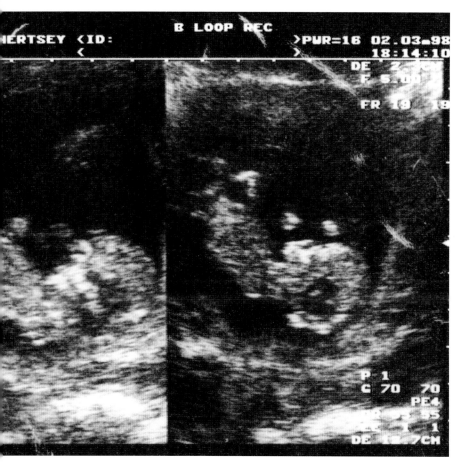

➤ Around 18-22 weeks of your pregnancy. This scan helps check all the different parts of your baby's body.

➤ You might be offered another scan later in your pregnancy, for example, to check the position of the placenta or to check the position of the baby.

Should I have a scan?

You don't have to have a scan but it might be useful to have one if:

• You want to see your baby before she is born.

• You are not sure when she might be born.

• You want to know if there is something seriously wrong with your baby.

Is the scan safe for the mother?

Having an ultrasound scan is easy, it does not hurt and it is safe for the mother.

Is it safe for the baby?

Researchers think that the scan is safe for the baby – they just have not been able to prove it. It seems certain that scans can't hurt your baby seriously, but more studies will need to be done before doctors can rule out the possibility that they could cause some kind of slight damage.

Will I be given a picture of my baby?

You may be given a photo of your baby to keep. Check with the hospital.

Will the scan be able to tell me if there are any problems?

The scan will be able to tell, for example, if your baby is not growing properly. But the scan will not be able to pick up *everything* that might be wrong with your baby. If the scan picks up a problem you will usually be offered other tests and you will be able to ask lots of questions.

How many scans will I be offered?

You will usually be offered two scans, depending on where you live:

➤ Before you are 18 weeks pregnant. You will usually have this scan quite early, by around 14 weeks. It helps work out when your baby will be born.

If I'm not happy with my maternity care, what can I do?

If you are concerned about the maternity care you are getting and want to discuss it, you can contact the Supervisor of Midwives for the Local Supervising Authority (LSA). They are available 24 hours a day, seven days a week. Ask your NHS Trust, maternity unit or midwife for contact details.

Anja's story

At my 12 week scan they measured the neck and the nose of the baby to calculate the risk of a baby with Down's syndrome. It took a very long time, and I was getting nervous, but in the end they told me that I only had a very small chance. But it spoilt the fun of seeing the baby a bit!

My 23 week scan was very nice, because the doctor explained everything I could see, and had time for my questions. It was difficult to lipread him, but he used a lot of gestures, and that was fine.

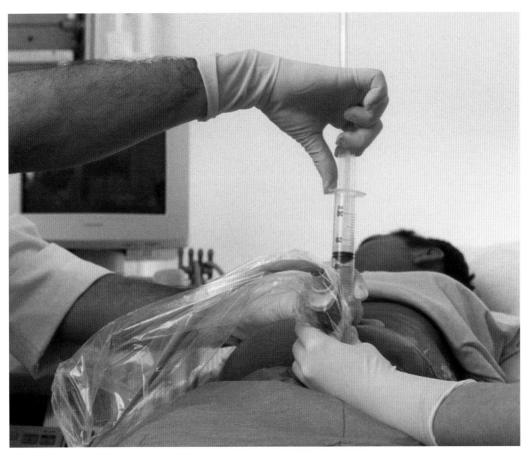

Amniocentesis is usually done by 20 weeks of pregnancy

Amniocentesis

What is this test for?

This is a **diagnostic** test. It is usually done by 20 weeks of pregnancy. It may be offered as early as 12 weeks. It is used to tell whether your baby may have some conditions such as Down's syndrome. You will need to wait up to four weeks for the test results and this can be a worrying time.

What does the test involve?

This test involves putting a long needle through the wall of your abdomen into the womb to remove some of your amniotic fluid. It is not usually painful but you can have a local anaesthetic to help make it less painful. You will have a scan at the same time so the doctor can see where your baby is.

Is the amniocentesis safe?

There is a less than 1% risk of miscarriage following the amniocentesis test. You should discuss the risk of this test with your GP and midwife before you agree to it.

Nuchal translucency test

What is this test for?

This is a **screening** test which you will be offered between 11 to 14 weeks. It is used to see how likely it is that your baby will have Down's syndrome and some other genetic conditions.

What does the test involve?

Babies in the womb have a thin layer of fluid between two folds of skin at the back of their neck. The nuchal translucency test involves measuring this fluid using an ultrasound scanner. If your baby appears to have a thicker layer of fluid you will be offered other tests to see whether she is more likely to have Down's syndrome and some other genetic conditions.

This is a new test, so it is not available on the NHS everywhere in the country. If you want to have it done privately, ask your GP for advice.

Chorionic villus sampling (CVS)

What is this test for?

This is a **diagnostic** test offered to women before they are 14 weeks pregnant. This test will be able to tell definitely whether your baby has a condition such as Down's Syndrome or some genetic conditions. You may be sent to a different hospital for CVS as not all hospitals can carry out this test.

What does the test involve?

A doctor will take a small sample of your placenta by putting a fine needle through your abdomen or cervix. The sample is sent away to a laboratory and you should receive the results within five to 10 days.

Is this test safe?

There is a 0.5 to 2% risk of miscarriage following the test. You should discuss this with your GP or midwife before agreeing to the test.

Can any of these tests show if my baby will be deaf or hearing?

None of the tests described in this chapter will be able to show whether your baby will be deaf or hearing before she is born. You will probably find out whether your baby is deaf or hearing shortly after she is born. Have a look at *Chapter 11 Your baby's first few days* for more information about Newborn Hearing Screening.

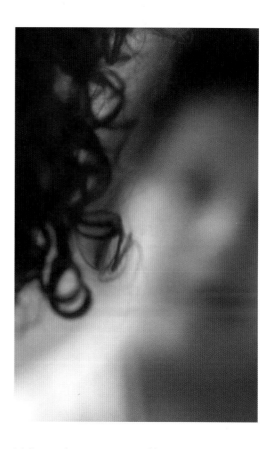

What happens if my test results show that something is wrong?

If your test results show that something is wrong with your baby you will be given lots of information and the chance to ask questions. You will usually be referred to an obstetrician – a doctor who specialises in birth. They should explain what is wrong with your baby and if you will need further tests. You will be given time to think about everything and to talk to your family, GP and midwife.

Try to find out as much as you can about what is wrong with your baby and how it may affect her after she is born. If tests show that there is something seriously wrong with your baby you may be unsure about whether you wish to carry on with the pregnancy. If you don't wish to carry on with the pregnancy your doctor will be able to tell you more about having a termination (also known as an abortion).

You may find it helpful to talk to someone who understands what you are going through – try contacting one of the organisations listed in Further information below for support and counselling.

Jennifer's story

At one of my scans for my eldest I wasn't able to get an interpreter so I asked the doctor to leave the lights on so that I could lipread her when she explained about the scan – she refused as it would make it hard for her to see the scan. So I made sure that I always had an interpreter at my other scans. Also it helped that I explained to them how to use the interpreters properly, for example, facing me when they talk.

Tips for talking to medical professionals

It can be difficult to talk to medical professionals especially if you are feeling stressed or worried. It may help to remember the following:

- **Benefits:** How will this treatment benefit my baby or me?
- **Risks:** Are there any risks to my baby or me?
- **Alternatives:** Are there any alternative treatments?
- **Intuition:** What is my gut feeling about what I want to do?
- **Nothing:** What will happen if we do nothing about this problem?

It may help you to ask:
- Is this an emergency or do we have time to talk?
- Who can give us a second opinion?
- How is our baby doing?

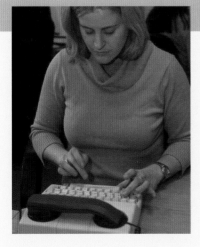

Further information

- Antenatal results and choices
- BLISS
- Contact a Family
- Marie Stopes International
- Mencap
- National Childbirth Trust

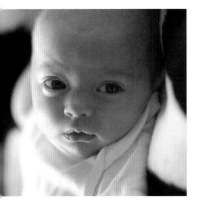

Chapter 8
If things go wrong during pregnancy

Most women go through pregnancy without any problems or complications but sometimes things can go wrong. You will usually have some warning signs so you will probably have time to get the best help available.

In this chapter we will look at the following complications:
- Vomiting.
- Anaemia.
- Bleeding.
- Miscarriage.
- Ectopic pregnancy.
- Placental abruption.
- Low-lying placenta.
- High blood pressure including:
  - Pregnancy-induced hypertension.
  - Pre-eclampsia.
  - Eclampsia.
  - Diabetes.

Vomiting
(see also the section on Morning sickness in *Chapter 5 How your body changes when you're pregnant*)

If you are vomiting (being sick) several times during the day and feel very ill, especially if this is after 14 weeks of pregnancy, you should contact your GP or midwife. You may need to be treated in hospital with a drip to give you fluids. You may also need to take medicine prescribed by your GP, until you can start drinking and eating again without being sick.

Anaemia

Some women develop anaemia during pregnancy. One type of anaemia is because your body doesn't have enough iron. Anaemia can make you feel tired and short of breath and you will have pale skin. Your GP can check to see if you are anaemic by giving you a blood test. If you are anaemic your GP may advise you to eat more food that is naturally rich in iron and to take iron tablets.

Bleeding

There are several possible reasons for bleeding including miscarriage, ectopic pregnancy, placental abruption or a low-lying placenta. We will look at all these in more detail below.

If you have any worries ...

If you are at all worried about your pregnancy or think there is anything wrong contact your GP or midwife. Find out the best way to contact them in an emergency.

If you have any bleeding

If you have any bleeding you should sit or lie down and call your midwife or GP immediately. If there is a lot of blood or you feel very faint, you may also need to call an ambulance, or the midwife or your GP will do this.

What is a miscarriage?

A miscarriage is also sometimes called 'spontaneous abortion'. If you lose a baby in the first 24 weeks of pregnancy this is known as a miscarriage. It is fairly common to have a miscarriage – at least one in 15 known pregnancies ends in miscarriage. Many women have a miscarriage without even realising they are pregnant. Most miscarriages occur in the first 12 weeks of pregnancy, but occasionally a woman will miscarry much later on in her pregnancy.

Are some women more likely to have a miscarriage than others?

Any pregnant woman can have a miscarriage, but you are more likely to have one if:
- You smoke.
- You have had more than one miscarriage already.
- You have certain medical conditions including fibroids, lupus or poorly controlled diabetes.
- You are older. The miscarriage rate doubles from age 20 to 40. At 40, about one-quarter of all pregnant women have a miscarriage.

What causes a miscarriage?

There are many different reasons why women have miscarriages:
- It seems that if there is something not right with your baby, such as abnormal chromosomes, you are more likely to have a miscarriage.
- A miscarriage can also happen if:
  - You have an infection.
  - Poorly controlled diabetes.
  - Problems with your thyroid.
  - Something wrong with your womb or cervix.
- Early in your pregnancy you may be offered two tests to check if there is a problem with your baby. These are

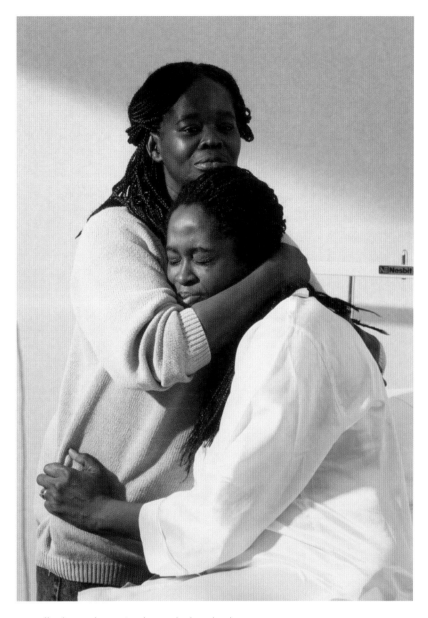

called amniocentesis and chrorionic villus sampling (CVS). These tests can cause a miscarriage in a very small number of women. There is more about these tests in *Chapter 7 Antenatal care*.

Help and advice

If you have had a miscarriage and would like to speak to someone about your feelings you might like to contact the Miscarriage Association, Stillbirth and Neonatal Death Society or The Foundation for the Study of Infant Deaths (See *Chapter 21 Further information* at the end of this book).

How do I know if I'm having a miscarriage?

If you are having a miscarriage you may have pains that feel like period pains and heavy bleeding which may include blood clots. However, you can have a miscarriage without even knowing you are having one, especially early in your pregnancy. Many women mistake a miscarriage for a late period. If you do start to bleed heavily call your GP immediately. You also need to rest.

Ectopic pregnancy

What is an ectopic pregnancy?

An ectopic pregnancy occurs when a fertilised egg starts growing outside the womb, generally in the fallopian tube. The fallopian tubes link your ovaries to your womb. It is a dangerous condition because, as the embryo grows, it starts to place pressure on the fallopian tube and surrounding organs in your body and the tube could bleed or burst. If an ectopic pregnancy is not removed it can lead to the death of the mother-to-be.

It is often difficult for your doctor to tell if you have an ectopic pregnancy. Some of the signs include:

- A low and sometimes strong pain on one side of your stomach.
- Bleeding from your vagina – this is often dark and watery.
- Pain when you go to the toilet.
- Pain in your shoulder tips (the ends of your shoulders).
- Fainting attacks.

If you have any of these signs, contact your GP immediately.

Can it be treated?

If your doctor thinks you have an ectopic pregnancy, you will need to go to hospital for a blood test, scan and a laparoscopy. This will help the doctor decide whether you definitely have an ectopic pregnancy. When you have a laparoscopy you will usually be given a general anaesthetic and a surgeon will insert a small tube with a light in it (this is the laparoscope) into a small cut near your tummy button. If you do have an ectopic pregnancy you will need treatment. This could involve surgery or drugs.

Sofia's story

At that time – three years ago, it was a bit of a wrong time really. It was around Christmas time that I found out I was pregnant. I was studying at college and working part-time and in the middle of the move to a new house. It was so stressful a time for me, really a wrong time for me to get pregnant. But we accepted it and went with the flow, even though it was really hard. I wasn't ready – but I just got on with it.

When I was three months pregnant everything seemed to be going well, then all of a sudden, I lost my baby. What happened was . . .

I was at my local hospital for my usual 20 week scan. I had booked an interpreter but there had been a last minute change and the social worker stepped in – she had BSL Level 3, I think*. When I had my scan, the nurse took a look at the screen and started to panic, saying that my baby was floating and she was finding it difficult to spot my baby on the computer as the computer was old. She left the room and said she would get a new computer.

Instantly, I knew something was not right. I hadn't felt right in the last two weeks. I had had a spot of bleeding two weeks ago but my GP had told me that all was fine and my baby's heartbeat was OK. She had told me to get plenty of rest.

But then the nurse came back, she told the interpreter that my baby's heart was not beating and that my baby had died. The interpreter became upset and told me "I'm so sorry" and then she started crying.

I couldn't work out what exactly was happening. I wasn't given any facts but from their expressions I could tell that something wasn't right. I asked the interpreter what was happening, then she told me that my baby had died and

I needed to give birth to it as soon as possible.

I was so shocked, I was not sure how to react. The interpreter tried holding my hand but I didn't want that, all I wanted was a clear translation. A qualified interpreter would have been neutral and factual but no, the interpreter, with me, was too emotional and I couldn't deal with it.

My partner, Ian, was at work. So I asked the nurse for a Minicom** as I wanted to speak to him. The nurse panicked, not knowing what a Minicom is, or where it was kept in the hospital. After a while, she found out that it was in the other building. I felt frustrated by the lack of deaf awareness. The interpreter offered me the use of her Minicom as she lived nearby. So I went with her and called Ian from her house. He was calm but upset. He came to the hospital straight from work and comforted me. It was a terrible experience.

After that, we were very upset and decided to take a break from everything. I went back to work and felt so emotional, I couldn't relax. It took me a long while to recover and move on with my life. Then we got married, and we decided to have a family – I am now five and half months pregnant! It took me by surprise – we planned to have a baby and tried for a long time! We had to use fertility treatment. It was a long process and hard work but it paid off. Instead of rushing around and being stressed like my first pregnancy Ian told me to take a complete rest and it worked!***

* BSL Level 3 is a qualification in British Sign Language. It does not include any interpreting skills.
** Minicom is a brand name for one particular make of textphone.
***Note from author – since Sofia told me her story she has given birth to a beautiful baby girl, and both are well.

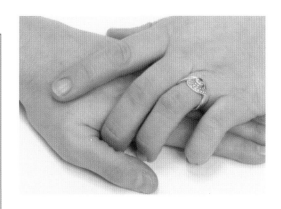

Will I be able to get pregnant again?
You are slightly less likely to get pregnant again if you have had an ectopic pregnancy but most women do get pregnant again.

Help and support if you lose a baby
If you have lost a baby through an ectopic pregnancy and would like to talk to someone about your feelings you can contact the Miscarriage Association.

Placental abruption

If you bleed after 24 weeks of pregnancy you may have a placental abruption. This happens when your placenta separates from the wall of your womb. This could be caused by:
- High blood pressure.
- A blow to your stomach.
- A fall.

You may also have pain at the same time as bleeding. You must go to hospital for treatment as soon as possible.

Low-lying placenta

Sometimes the placenta develops too low in the womb. This is known as a low-lying placenta. Bleeding happens when the cervix starts to get ready for labour. An ultrasound scan usually picks this up.

If this happens, you will have to go to hospital for the rest of your pregnancy. Sometimes you will need to have a caesarean section, as it may be too dangerous for you or the baby, if you have a vaginal birth.

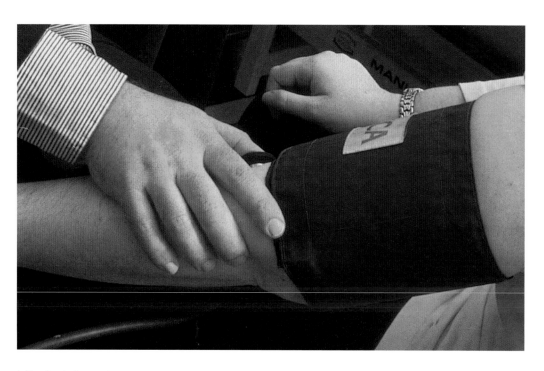

High blood pressure

The following conditions are linked to pregnancy.
- Pregnancy induced hypertension.
- Pre-eclampsia.
- Eclampsia.

Pregnancy induced hypertension
Your blood pressure will be checked at every antenatal visit. It usually stays similar to your normal blood pressure but sometimes it is raised in the later stages of pregnancy. If it is too high it means that your baby might get less oxygen. Some women already have high blood pressure before they get pregnant.

If the high blood pressure is caused by your pregnancy it is known as **pregnancy induced hypertension** and you may be given medication.

If your blood pressure is always high you'll probably be advised to rest.

Pre-eclampsia
What is pre-eclampsia?
Pre-eclampsia is a disease that affects the placenta. It develops after 20 weeks of pregnancy and is more common if you are pregnant with your first baby and in women with a family history of the disease. The symptoms include:
- High blood pressure.
- Protein in the urine.
- Sometimes, your hands, feet and face will be swollen.

It is possible to have pre-eclampsia and feel perfectly well. This is why your blood pressure is checked at every antenatal visit. Tell the midwife if you think you have swollen hands, feet or ankles. However, pre-eclampsia can get worse very suddenly, causing severe problems for you and your baby. If this happens you might get severe headaches, have problems with your eyesight, such as seeing flashing lights, and pain in your upper stomach. You might have an epileptic-type seizure (fit). This condition is called **eclampsia** and you will need immediate care.

Farah's story

Though I speak well for myself, I am still Deaf. My midwife has often told me that to book an appointment, I could just call her on the phone as I speak well. I explained that I can't hear the phone and prefer to use a fax, for ease of communication, knowing that they are not aware of Typetalk.* She hesitated, saying that it would be difficult as the fax machine is held in a different office and there is no guarantee they will check my fax.

This is also a problem at my GP's surgery. Once I used my fax to book an appointment with my GP and he was annoyed at the number of faxes sent between us and told me to get my hearing husband to arrange the appointment for me. Why should I? I am a very independent person and want to do things for myself.

*RNID Typetalk is a national telephone relay service.

How is pre-eclampsia treated?

If your midwife or GP thinks that you have pre-eclampsia, you will probably have to go to hospital to be closely monitored in case things suddenly get worse. The only treatment for pre-eclampsia is for your baby to be born. This may be a problem if you are still early in your pregnancy. The risks to you and your baby from continuing the pregnancy with pre-eclampsia have to be carefully weighed against the risks to the baby of being born early.

Diabetes in pregnancy

Some women develop diabetes, which is related to pregnancy. This is known as **gestational diabetes**. It means that you have a high level of sugar in your blood. It doesn't usually last and it won't necessarily harm your baby. In most cases, it goes shortly after your baby is born but it may be a sign that you will develop diabetes later in life.

Your urine (wee) will be tested for sugar at each antenatal visit. If your GP or midwife finds sugar you will then be offered other tests. You will be referred to a specialist diabetic consultant doctor, a dietician and a consultant obstetrician. You may have to take a drug called insulin. The specialists will help your GP and midwife to check your health and your baby's health carefully for the rest of your pregnancy and labour.

After the baby is born you will be checked to see if the diabetes has gone.

Other medical conditions

If you have a medical condition you must talk to your GP and/or midwife. The consultant obstetrician will usually need to see you and you may need to see a medical specialist.

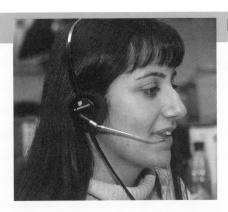

Further information

- www.babycentre.co.uk
- National Childbirth Trust
- Miscarriage Association
- Stillbirth and Neonatal Death Society

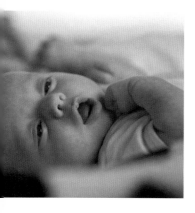

Chapter 9

Choosing where, and how, to have your baby

What is a birth plan?

Many women find it helpful to prepare a birth plan when they are pregnant. A birth plan is when you write down what you would like to happen during labour and your baby's birth. Your midwife uses it to know what you want. You can talk about it with your midwife, friends, partner and your birth companion but it's up to you what you write in the plan.

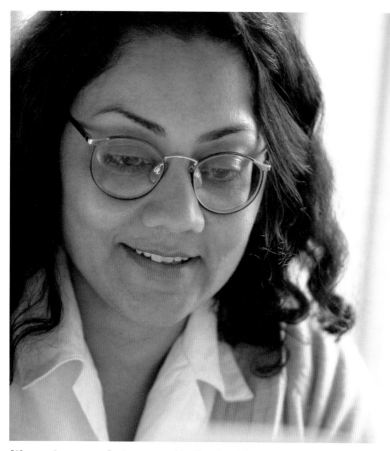

It's up to you what you write in the birth plan

A birth companion is also known as a labour companion. This is someone you can choose to support you during birth. It could be your partner, mother, sister, friend or anyone else you trust and feel comfortable with.

Some women choose to get help from a specially trained 'doula'. This is a woman who has learned how to give particular support to women when they are giving birth.

A birth plan might cover:
- Who you want with you during labour and birth.
- What pain relief you want.
- Which positions you might want to try during labour and birth.
- How you feel about medical procedures being used to speed up labour and birth.
- If you mind having midwifery students present.
- What you want to do immediately after your baby has been born, for example, do you want your new baby put on your tummy so you can hold her and she might start sucking at your breast?
- If you want your baby to be given Vitamin K (see *Chapter 11 Your baby's first few days*).
- The importance of having everything clearly explained to you.
- Your needs as a deaf woman and how you prefer to communicate. This can help ensure that all midwives and staff you come into contact with are aware that you are deaf and can explain everything clearly to you.

- Whether you want an interpreter to be present throughout the labour and birth. Do you want the interpreter to remain throughout the birth or leave the room to give you and your partner the space to share the special moment with your baby?
- Whether you want a female interpreter.
- Where you want the interpreter to sit or stand in the room.
- How you want to communicate with the midwife and other staff if you don't want an interpreter for the labour and birth. For example, you can agree some basic signs so that you can understand each other.
- What you want to happen if there is an emergency and you can't get an interpreter at short notice. Do you want information written down on paper? Do you want clear face-to-face communication so you can lipread? Do you want to use gestures if necessary?

However much you plan, it is important to stress that no labour or birth is the same so it is difficult to know or plan ahead what will happen. While a birth plan is a good way of making sure your midwife knows what you want from your labour and birth, you may find that the plan is never used.

Choosing where to have your baby

You can choose whether to have your baby at home, in a GP/midwife unit or in a hospital, although this may vary depending on where you live. It is your choice where you have your baby. To help you make that choice you can ask your GP or midwife lots of questions.

Choosing a hospital birth

You may be able to choose which hospital you want to have your baby in, if there is more than one in your area. To help you make your decision you can visit the hospital and find out:

- Is it all right for you to eat and drink as you please during labour, or will you only be allowed water?

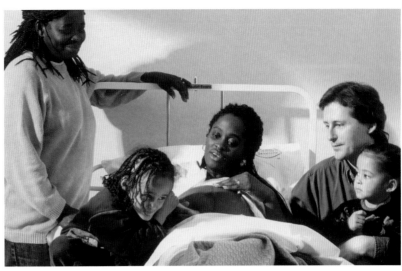

You can choose whether to have a baby at home, in a GP/midwife unit or in a hospital

- Can you wear your own clothes for labour?
- How many people can you bring with you to support you during labour?
- Is there a birthing pool and midwives experienced in using it?
- Will it be possible to have an epidural at any time, or only during certain hours?
- Can you give birth in any position you choose?
- How long will you stay in hospital after the birth?
- What are the visiting hours? Can your partner and other children visit you outside these hours?
- Is there a textphone available?
- Are staff deaf aware?
- What communication support will be available?

Elizabeth's story

I put in big capitals on my birth plan that I was hard of hearing and how they could help me. I think that helped a bit, but when the crunch came, nobody told me what was going on. I was cut when I didn't want to be and I did feel ignored. But this may have not been because I am hard of hearing – even hearing mothers can feel like this at birth. When the baby was born, they told my husband it was a baby girl – and I was lying on the bed, exhausted and forever asking whether I had a baby boy or a girl while the midwife and the nurse were cleaning my baby. The midwife was stern and told me that I had a girl. That midwife came on shift while I was in labour so she wasn't aware that I am hard of hearing.

Anja's story

I had a tour of the maternity ward. I had to phone a couple of times beforehand to make sure that the hospital got me an interpreter. I went, and it turned out that they had booked a communication support worker, who had only Level 2*. Worse still, it was someone who didn't have any experience with childbirth, so he didn't have a clue what all the terms were about.

*BSL Level 2 is a qualification in British Sign Language. It does not include any interpreting skills.

What are the advantages?
- You can choose any type of pain relief including an epidural – a particular type of pain relief. See *Chapter 10 Labour and birth.*
- If there are problems, everything you need will be in the hospital so you shouldn't have to move, for example, to another hospital.

What are the disadvantages?
- You are more likely to be monitored by electronic machinery.
- You may be more likely to have a drip (if you have an epidural you will also need a drip in your arm).

Rosie's story

I remember vividly a tour of the maternity ward. Sam and I turned up and there were 30 couples with us. We found out no sign language interpreter was booked because the tour happens every Sunday and it is open to all. I mentioned to the midwife that Sam and I are deaf and need clear communication, for example, good face contact for clear lipreading, and good lighting, but we missed out everything that was said. I was frustrated, as we wanted to know what to expect and to be able to ask questions.

And because of our experiences of the maternity ward tour, Sam and I agreed to establish a clear rule of communication, especially during labour. (See *Chapter 10 Labour and birth* for Rosie's story about using a clear rule for communication).

Choosing a home birth

If you would like a home birth talk it over with your GP or midwife. Some people are concerned that home births are not as safe as hospital births but research suggests that home birth is just as safe as a hospital birth if there are no complications with your pregnancy.

What are the advantages?
- You might feel more in control and more relaxed.
- You will have familiar things around you and you can wander around freely.
- You might prefer a home birth if you don't like hospitals.
- You might like the idea of being more private in your own home.

What are the disadvantages?
- You may feel safer in hospital with easy access to specialist medical care and some types of pain relief such as an epidural.
- Even if you choose a home birth, if something goes wrong you may need to go to hospital either before, during, or after your labour. If you do have to go into hospital, your midwife will go with you but may not be able to deliver your baby.

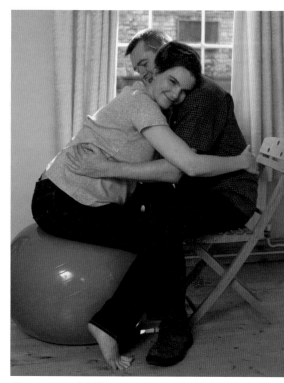

If you would like a home birth talk it over with your GP or midwife

Choosing a GP or midwife unit

A GP or midwife unit might be a separate unit or part of a hospital's ordinary maternity ward. You may prefer to have a baby in one of these units, because the same midwife who has been with you throughout your pregnancy may be able to stay with you during labour and birth. Your GP or midwife will generally only recommend that you have your baby in a GP or midwife unit if you are likely to have no complications at birth.

Katie's story

I did not have an interpreter during the birth. I decided I would manage as long as I had my hearing aids and my husband was present. The staff spoke clearly, although some had to be reminded to look at me directly. My husband would repeat if he thought I had missed anything.

Anja's story

My first two children were born at hospital, but I gave birth at home to my third one. I liked it so much more than in hospital. In the hospital I saw so many different nurses, midwives and doctors, and I had to explain over and over again about my deafness, the history of my deafness, and communication. At home we only saw one midwife, and it was very relaxed.

Janet's story

A midwifery-led birth centre was what we originally wanted, but there was none in our area apart from private clinics. So it was either the hospital or our home. We decided for a home birth as I wanted to feel comfortable and relaxed during the labour. We prepared for our home birth by reading books and looking up a few discussion lists on the Internet. With that, we felt confident that we could cope with any difficulty during the labour.

We told our friends and acquaintances that we wanted a home birth. Most told us it would be safer at the hospital, however I still wanted a home birth. My husband supported me in my choices.

Because we asked for a home birth, I had two midwives looking after me during the whole labour – even after we transferred to the hospital.

Communication support

Before you make your choice about where you want to have your baby you should discuss what communication support will be available at home, in hospital or in a GP or midwife unit. You might want to ask:

- If I choose a home birth but have to go to hospital at short notice what is the chance of there being an interpreter there for me?
- Will my midwife book an interpreter if I have a home birth?
- If the interpreter fails to turn up at home, or in hospital, what alternative communication support will be available, to ensure that I understand what is happening?
- How long will an interpreter be able to stay with me after the birth?

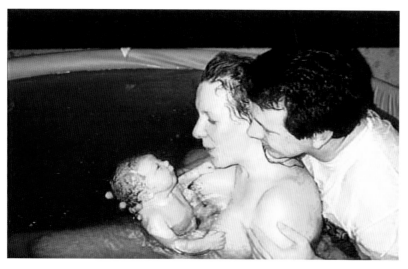

Some women choose to use a birthing pool

Sharon's story

I had a midwife with BSL Level 2* for my first labour which took place in hospital. As I had a very long labour she eventually had to end her shift and I then had a midwife with a strong accent during the actual birth.** Due to the drip I was well 'out of it' and could only understand my Deaf husband, Jason. Every time the midwife said "push", by the time Jason lipread and interpreted for me, it was too late to push so in the end I just shut my eyes and let my instincts guide me and push whenever I felt the urge. A few pushes later, my beautiful baby boy was born.

*BSL Level 2 is a qualification in British Sign Language. It does not include any interpreting skills.
**Lipreading someone with an unfamiliar accent can be difficult.

Waterbirths

Some women choose to use a birthing pool for their labour and occasionally to give birth.

- You can hire a birthing pool if you are planning to have your baby at home. Contact the National Childbirth Trust or the Active Birth Centre for help and advice.
- If you are going to have your baby in hospital, check to see if you can use a birthing pool and if it will be available when you need it. If the hospital does not have one, they may be happy for you to hire one and bring it in.
- Check if there is a midwife who knows how to support women using a birthing pool.
- You may be able to go to waterbirth classes at the hospital.

For more information about waterbirths and using a birthing pool contact:

- The Association for Improvements in the Maternity Services.
- National Childbirth Trust.
- Also see our *Chapter 10 Labour and birth*.

If you have problems getting your choice of birthplace organised you could ask to talk to the Supervisor of Midwives.

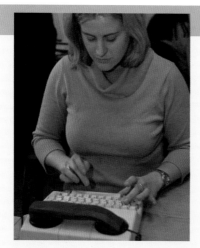

Further information

- The Association for Improvements in the Maternity Services
- www.birthchoiceuk.com
- Midwives Information and Resource Service
- National Childbirth Trust

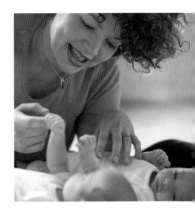

Chapter 10
Labour and birth

It is a good idea to ask other mothers and your midwife about labour and birth. However, everyone's experience of labour and birth is different.

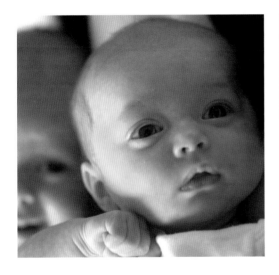

Going into labour

Labour happens in three stages.

First stage

Contractions open up the cervix. They are weak and irregular at first, then they become stronger and more regular. First stage can take several hours and can be divided into two stages – 'early first stage' and 'later first stage'.

- **Early first stage**
  It may take six to eight hours for the cervix to dilate (get wider) to 3-4cm, for mothers having their first baby.

- **Later first stage**
  Once the cervix is as wide as 3-4 cm, it can take another six to eight hours, or more, to be fully dilated to 10cm. During this time contractions get stronger and more frequent. Sometimes, near the end of this stage, the contractions ease off for a short time.

Second stage

Once the cervix is dilated it may take an hour or so, before you feel a real urge to push. This stage usually takes longer for first time mothers, but varies a lot. Your baby is born in this stage.

Third stage

After your baby has been born your placenta comes out of your womb. This stage can last from a few minutes to over an hour.

Julie's story

My mum and husband were there during the birth. I spent the weekend at the hospital as my blood pressure was a bit high and they wanted to keep me in for observation. My labour started early. I was getting scared because of the contractions and I couldn't believe how bad the pain was. Thankfully I had some pain relief during the labour.

The midwife accepted my mum's presence as they knew I needed help with communication because I was under pain relief. The only negative part of the birth was that when my mum came to help me when I was in labour, they made her wait outside for two hours because it was outside official visiting hours. If I wanted to talk to her, I had to sit outside in the corridor from the ward. The senior midwife wasn't happy when she found out and told me that my mum had a right to be with me and she apologised to me.

I was happy and over the moon to have my newborn son with me after a nine month wait. I couldn't believe it when I saw him and cuddled him, thinking, "wow, I created a little human being who grew in my bump".

How will I know if I've gone into labour?

There are several signs to look out for.

- **A show**
  This is when the plug of mucus that has formed in the neck of your womb during pregnancy, comes away. The mucus will look like clear jelly, or may be pink, if it is stained with blood. You can have a show several days before labour starts.

- **Contractions**
  This is when your womb tightens up and then lets go. This may happen as often as every two minutes but early in labour it is more likely to be every 20 to 30 minutes. Early contractions may just feel like backache but if you put your hand on your bump you may feel your womb hardening. Contractions usually get longer, stronger and closer together nearer to the birth. They are usually regular. Contractions build up and fade away.

- **Waters breaking**
  'Waters' is the word given to the liquid that surrounds your baby in the womb. Waters don't always break at the start of labour. If they do, they may gush out or just be a trickle. If you think your waters have broken you need to contact the midwife or hospital.

  You may also have frequent bowel movements, this means you will be having a poo more often.

  You may also just feel different.

When should I call the midwife, or go to the GP/midwife unit or hospital?

Call your midwife or go to hospital (although it is a good idea to tell them you are coming first):
- When you think you are in active labour.
- When you start to feel that it would help you relax if midwives were there to help you.
- If you want to use pain relief that is not available at home.
- If your waters break with a gush.
- If you have a question about what is normal or need reassurance.

What is the role of the midwife?
Your midwife is there to:
- Help you give birth safely and to support you.
- Tell you when you're doing things right.
- Encourage you, and comfort you and your birth partner.

You need to be aware that if you are having your baby in hospital, the same midwife may not be able to stay with you the whole time.

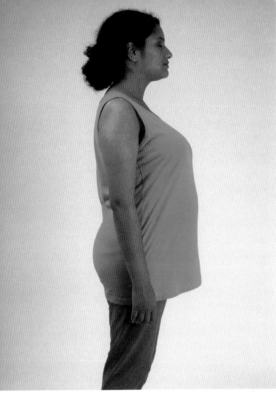

Nearly all women find that being upright helps them to cope better than lying down

First stage of labour

During the first stage of labour your contractions will start to push your baby's head down onto your cervix. As the cervix opens up, your baby's head will start to move into your pelvis. Contractions will usually last for 20 to 40 seconds. During this stage they will also start to get closer together, and stronger, for example you may get them every two to seven minutes. You will feel pain mainly in your lower back, tummy and hips.

Getting help with the pain of labour

There are many ways of managing the pain of labour.
- Some methods involve relaxing and 'working with the pain' so that you can use your body's own way of coping with pain.
- Other methods use drugs to stop, or reduce, the pain.

Using natural methods to relieve pain

Using breathing
It is a good idea to learn breathing techniques in antenatal classes. It is best to breathe steadily throughout your contractions. Breathe in through your nose and out gently through your mouth. Concentrate particularly as you breathe out.

Keep focusing on breathing in through your nose and blowing out gently through your mouth. Even the longest contraction will only last 90 seconds. Your breathing can help you cope with each contraction, one at a time. In between contractions, simply rest.

Create a picture in your mind

This is often known as 'visualisation'.
- Some women find it helpful to picture what is happening as they give birth. You could try to picture your baby moving down and being born.
- Or you could try viewing the pain as a spot of colour that changes colour each time you breathe in.
- Or try focusing on something bright, then close your eyes and keep the picture as clear as possible. Concentrate on keeping it clear until you have to open your eyes and refocus again.
- You may prefer to picture yourself in a favourite place – thinking about pleasant things can help your body relax.

Make sure you are comfortable
Being comfortable in labour will really help you cope with the pain.
- Early in your labour you may feel that you are able to manage your contractions on your own. It may be enough just to get into the position that helps you the most and makes you feel comfortable.

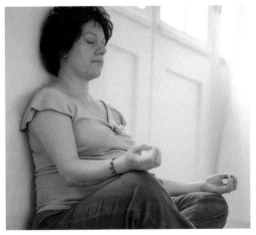

Create a picture in your mind and try to relax

- Nearly all women find that being upright helps them to cope better than lying down. Try walking around as much as you can.
- You will probably find it helps if you lean forward. Try leaning against the back of a chair, or on to the hospital bed. You may want to kneel and lean on to a chair. If you have backache, try going on all fours. You can use a bean bag or lots of pillows under your knees and hands to make yourself comfortable. Leaning forward widens the space between your back and the front of your pelvis, giving your baby more room. It also helps relieve pressure on your back.
- If you keep your knees apart this helps your pelvis to open up and gives your baby more room.
- If you're standing upright, you might find it comforting to rock round and round from the waist, and forwards and backwards.
- Ask your midwife or birth partner to remind you to move around if you want to.
- Above all do what feels right for your body.

Try massage

You might find it helps with pain if someone massages the lower part of your back when you are having contractions – however, you might not want to be touched at all! It is a good idea to practise with your birth partner before you go into labour.

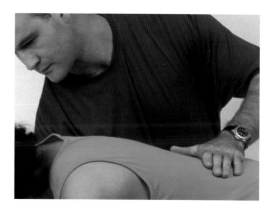

Taking a bath or shower

Lots of women find that warm water can give a lot of pain relief. You can either take a shower or a bath. Try sitting on a plastic chair or an upturned plastic bucket if you are in the shower.
You might find it helps to kneel on all fours in a full bath.

Using a birthing pool

Many women like to use a birthing pool. Some use it just for the first stage of labour and others stay in for the second stage to give birth. They find the water supports them and lets them move freely and they may not need pain relief. Some studies show that you are less likely to need a forceps or ventouse delivery if you spend some time in water (see later in this chapter). A birthing pool can also be helpful if you have any kind of physical disability.

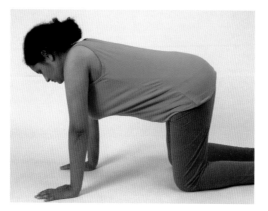

Massage guidelines for birth partners

- **Make sure *you* are relaxed.**
- **Make sure your hands are warm – if they're cold or sticky run them under the hot water tap.**
- **Use just a small amount of vegetable oil, for example, olive oil.**
- **Try to massage your partner slowly, and build up a regular rhythm.**
- **Always check that you are giving the massage in the right part of your partner's body and that she finds it comfortable. You may want to try her lower back.**

TENS

What is TENS?

TENS = transcutaneous electrical nerve stimulation. A TENS machine gives out small pulses that block the pain messages being sent to the brain during labour and encourages your body to produce endorphins – natural pain killing substances found in the nervous system.

How does TENS work?

A TENS machine has a small box you can fit in your pocket. Wires come out of the box and connect to two pairs of electrodes. These are stuck onto your back using sticky pads. You can use a dial and a button to control the number of pulses given out by the machine.

TENS works best if you try it out during the last weeks of pregnancy and then use it from the start of labour. You will need to hire

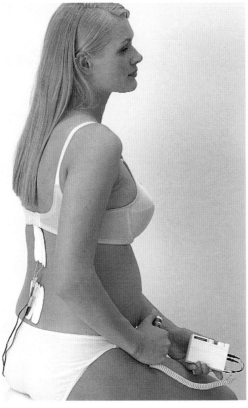

a unit so that you can practise using it before labour starts. Machines cost about £30 to hire but some hospitals hire them for free. You may have to pay for the sticky pads. Many hospitals also run a class to show you where to put the electrodes and how to get the best out of the machine.

Most women find TENS simple to use but not everyone finds it effective. You can use it with other forms of pain relief.

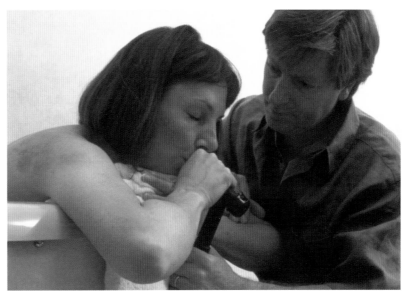

You may find it helpful to use gas and air to help you manage your pain

Using drugs to control pain

Using gas and air

You may find it helpful to use gas and air to help you manage your pain. The gas is a mixture of oxygen and nitrous oxide and is often called entonox. You will have to breathe the gas and air in through a mouthpiece or a facemask. If you are having a home birth the midwife will bring a gas cylinder to your house. Gas and air usually work well but it is only a mild pain killer and some women find it makes them feel sick.

How to use gas and air

- Put the mouthpiece into your mouth at the very beginning of your contraction and breathe deeply and evenly. This will make the valve work.
- It takes about 20 seconds for the gas to build up in your bloodstream and to reduce your pain. As the contraction fades away, remove the mouthpiece and just breathe normally until you feel the next contraction starting.
- If you use it as soon as you feel a contraction coming, it will help reduce the pain by the time the contraction is really strong.
- The gas will make you feel a little light-headed during the contraction but by the end of the contraction, your head will have cleared.
- You should hold the mask or mouthpiece yourself. If someone holds the mask for you, you may breathe in more gas than you want.

Pethidine
What is pethidine?

Pethidine is an opiate – a drug that acts as a sedative and works by changing the way you feel about your pain. Pethidine can be used if you are having a home birth.

If you have a long, tiring labour, pethidine can help by giving you the chance to rest, or even sleep. However it may make you feel sick and you won't be able to move about after having it. It is usually given with another drug to stop you from being sick.

How do I take pethidine?

- The midwife will inject pethidine into your thigh or bottom. You will need to lie down if you have pethidine, as you are likely to feel sleepy once it takes effect.
- An injection of pethidine lasts about three to four hours. You should not be given pethidine when you are close to giving birth because it can make your baby sleepy and cause breathing problems.

Epidurals
What is an epidural?

An epidural involves giving you a drug – a local anaesthetic. It stops you feeling anything from the waist down including the pain of your contractions. An epidural has to be given by an anaesthetist in hospital so you can't have one if you are having a home birth.

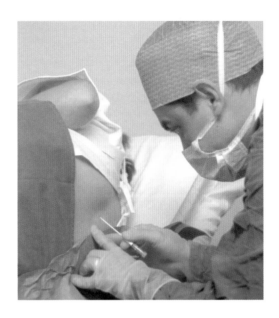

Many women don't feel any pain when they have an epidural. You will have a drip in your hand before the epidural is started. Once you have an epidural your blood pressure, contractions and your baby's heartbeat will be monitored.

Unless your hospital can offer you a mobile epidural, you will have to remain on the bed and are more likely to require forceps or ventouse to deliver your baby.

How does an epidural work?

There are different ways that you can be given an epidural:

- The epidural gets into your body via a fine hollow tube – known as a catheter – which is inserted into your lower back. The epidural lasts for about two to four hours but can be 'topped up' through the tube.
- A mobile epidural involves the same procedure, but the end of the catheter is attached to a pump. This usually pumps a small amount of anaesthetic and an opiate (another type of drug, which relieves pain) at regular intervals. As the dose is low you may be able to move about, and then push down in the second stage of labour.
- You are first injected with an anaesthetic in the base of your spine. This gives a couple of hours of pain relief. At the same time an epidural catheter is also put in position. Once the pain relief from the injection has worn off you can then have a traditional epidural.

Rosie's story

I decided to have an epidural. I had written down in my birth plan that if the pain got worse then I wanted to have an epidural. We had set up a communication rule from the beginning and that came in useful, especially when I was having the epidural. I was told that I must not move while having the injection but it was difficult because when the contraction came, I had to move. So Sam and I agreed, that while the epidural was taking place, if I had a contraction, I would tell Sam. Sam would then say 'stop' to the anaesthetist who was behind me, to stop them putting the epidural into my spine until the contraction stopped. That worked very well.

What is an induced birth?

An induced birth means you are given help to start your labour. This may be because:

- You are 10 days or more past the date your baby is due to be born.
- You have pre-eclampsia. We tell you more about this in *Chapter 8 If things go wrong during pregnancy*.
- Your baby is not growing well.
- Your waters have broken, but after 72 hours, you are still not having contractions.
- You have diabetes.

How is labour induced?

There are three main ways of starting labour:

- Prostaglandin pessaries or gel. These are placed in your vagina.
- Your waters will be broken.
- A drip is used to give you a drug called syntocinon.

There are some risks involved with having an induced labour and your doctor should tell you about these.

How will I be monitored?

- If you have a drip you will usually have to stay in bed and your midwife will monitor your baby's heartbeat constantly.
- If you have had pessaries or your waters have been broken, you won't need to stay in bed all the time. Your baby's heartbeat will be monitored, but not all the time.

Second stage of labour

During the second stage of labour your baby is actually born.

- While her head is coming out you may feel a hot sensation between your legs.
- Your baby's shoulders and body are generally born in a single contraction after her head.
- You will find it easier to push if you try kneeling or squatting with help from your birth partner and the midwife. Or try leaning on a bed, or side of a pool if you are having a waterbirth. Your midwife may suggest that you try to concentrate on 'breathing' your baby out.

Rosie and Sam's story

Rosie

I had pre-eclampsia two weeks prior to birth. My blood pressure was normal throughout my pregnancy but when I went to my next appointment with my GP, a few days after I left work, it took us by surprise to find that my blood pressure was so high. I had to stay in the hospital for a few days. I was told that I had pre-eclampsia and would need to be induced.

When I was induced, the midwife put a special gel into my vagina. The aim of the gel was to make my body think it was ready for labour. I found it hard to lipread the midwife because it was night and the lighting was not very good. The midwife was so nice and made gestures that all would be fine. That happened about 11 o'clock at night. My husband Sam was with me at the time. They hoped for my labour to start sometime on the following morning and then told Sam that he had to go home. I was upset as I wanted him by my side through the night.

Sam

Before I left, I had a long chat with the midwife and explained to her the importance of contacting me if Rosie went into labour during the night. I gave the midwife all my contact details, Minicom, fax, SMS, everything. She said she couldn't fax me as the fax machine was in the other building. I remained firm and insisted that the best way for her to contact me was by fax and constantly asked her if she understood me. I was really insistent as I felt it was very important for me to be there for Rosie for labour and I didn't want to miss out on anything.

Rosie

I slept through the night but the pain of being induced was a bit like a heavy period pain. Sam came that morning at nine o'clock to be with me. I was taken to the labour room and the doctor broke my waters by inserting a hook inside me. The water was warm and rippled down my legs.

I then focused on the second stage of birth which took about half an hour. Sam and the midwife were very encouraging and told me to push. I didn't feel anything even though I was pushing. I wasn't sure but the midwife told me I was doing very well.

What really hit me the most was the use of a mirror. The midwife asked me if I wanted to see my baby. Obviously, I couldn't see because of my bump, but then the midwife showed me through the mirror. It was WOW, it really hit me that I was really having a baby and that helped me a lot to push and give birth. Sam was busy, helping me with my breathing, as well as taking pictures and a video of the special moment for us to treasure. The baby was then born, the head was the hardest part but the body followed out so quickly that Sam missed it.

So I would recommend to any deaf parents – have your mirror handy, it is definitely worth it!

- When your baby's head is ready to come out your midwife will tell you to pant, rather than push, so that the baby's head can come out slowly.
- For some women this is a really hard time. It can take a lot of effort and hard work. Try to work with the midwife and use your body to help you give birth to your baby.

You may want to plan more carefully for the second stage of labour. It is worth having a practice beforehand and thinking about how you want to communicate. Stick to instructions that you can understand immediately such as 'push', 'don't push' or 'pant'.

Will instruments be used to help deliver my baby?

Sometimes medical staff might need to use instruments to help you deliver your baby. There are two sorts – forceps and ventouse.

These might be needed if:
- You have been pushing for a long time.
- You are exhausted.
- Your baby's heartbeat shows signs of distress.

What are forceps?

Forceps look like stainless steel salad servers. Your midwife will help you put your legs up in stirrups and the doctor will make a cut through the back of your vagina to enlarge the opening. This is known as an episiotomy. The forceps will then be placed gently round your baby's head. When you have your next contraction, you push and your doctor pulls your baby out.

What is a ventouse?

A ventouse looks like a small plastic cup. Suction is used to help the cup stick to your baby's head and to help pull your baby out. You probably won't need an episiotomy for a ventouse delivery.

What is a caesarean section?

A caesarean section is an operation to deliver your baby.

What is a planned caesarean?

If you and your obstetrician think you should have a planned caesarean you will be given a date for you to go into hospital before you go into labour. This means you will know in advance that you will be having a caesarean. It is also known as an elective caesarean.

You might need a caesarean section because:
- Your placenta is 'low-lying' and is blocking the way for your baby to come out of your vagina.
- Your baby is too big compared to your pelvis and it would be difficult for your baby to born through the vagina.
- Your baby isn't growing properly.
- You have a serious medical condition.
- You have a breech baby (see later in this chapter).

What is an unplanned caesarean?

If you have a caesarean during labour this is known as an unplanned or emergency caesarean. There are various reasons why you might need this. The decision to operate on you might happen quite quickly.

What happens during a caesarean?

Before the operation, you will have to:
- Sign a consent form.
- Remove your jewellery.
- Take out your contact lenses, false teeth and hairgrips.
- Drink some medicine. This will help make the acid in your stomach less acidic.
- Remove nail varnish. Pale nails can be a sign of low oxygen levels in your

blood so you need to remove nail varnish so that your nails can be checked.

If you wear hearing aids you will only have to remove them when you have been given an anaesthetic.

During the operation:
- There will be around eight doctors, midwives and other staff helping at your caesarean.
- You might have some of your pubic hair shaved off - the hair around your vagina.
- A drip will be put into your arm.
- A catheter will be put into your bladder. This is a tube which empties your bladder.
- Heart monitors will be fixed to your chest.
- You will either be given a local anaesthetic, which means that you'll be awake for the operation, or a general anaesthetic which means you will sleep through the caesarean. If you are awake you won't feel any pain.
- The surgeon will make a cut about six inches long, along your bikini line (where the waistband of your bikini bottoms would be). If you are awake you won't be able to see anything because there will be a screen across your chest, below your shoulders.
- Your partner will be able to stay with you, if you want, but usually only if you have had a local anaesthetic and are awake yourself.
- Once the operation starts it will take about 10 minutes to deliver your baby. After she has been born she will be checked to see if she is OK and then you will be able to cuddle her while your operation is completed.
- The whole operation takes about 40 minutes.

After your caesarean

- You will find that it will take you longer to recover than women who have given birth vaginally. You will be in pain after the operation and will be given pain relief. Your catheter may be left in for 24 hours and your drip may stay in for one to two days.

- You may need iron tablets.
- The surgery may make it difficult for you to stand upright at first but you will be encouraged to get up and move around.
- You shouldn't lift anything heavier than your baby for about six weeks.
- You won't be able to drive for about six weeks, but you should check with your insurance company.

Third stage of labour

This is when the placenta or afterbirth comes away from the womb and passes out through your vagina. It is possible to have a 'natural' third stage if you have had a normal labour. This is when the midwife lets your placenta come out without any help. It can take between 10 minutes to an hour.

However, many midwives prefer to help deliver the placenta. Your midwife will inject a drug, usually syntometrine, into your thigh, to help the placenta come out of your vagina. This means the placenta comes out about seven minutes after you have given birth.

While this stage is happening you could be holding your baby. You may be encouraged to hold her 'skin-to-skin'. This means she is placed naked on you, but you are both covered to keep you warm. Most babies are ready to breastfeed within an hour of being born and the midwife will be able to help you. You should discuss what type of third stage labour you want and decide with the midwife what would be best for you.

Farah's story

I was worried about the birth. My due date had passed and my baby wouldn't come out. Finally I went into labour. Also because I was overdue, I asked for a caesarean because I felt that it would be a suitable option as my baby was too big. However the doctor thought otherwise and insisted that I should keep trying for a natural delivery. I thought it would be impossible as I felt so huge, and it would create too much pain for me to go through.

However, no matter how hard I tried, the baby became distressed and I was given an emergency caesarean. My son was born and measured 56cm long – he looked older as if he was one or two months old already!

What is a breech baby?

Most babies move so that their head is facing down in the womb during the last few months of pregnancy. If your baby's head stays up, instead of down, you have what is known as a 'breech baby'. If you have a breech baby your GP or midwife will discuss the different options available to you. These include:

- Waiting to see if your baby turns round on her own in the last few weeks.
- Having the baby turned by a doctor who pushes her round gently from outside your womb. This is called ECV or external cephalic version.
- A caesarean section.

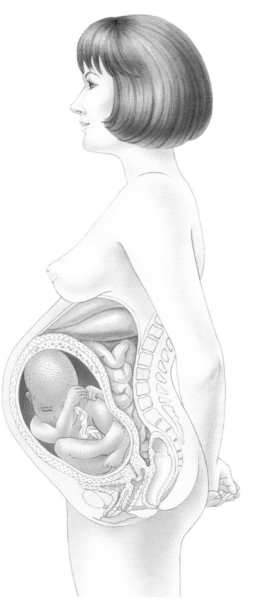

If you have a breech baby your GP or midwife will discuss the different options available to you

Patricia's story

I had a good pregnancy. I had always planned for a home birth and wanted to have as much of a natural birth as possible.

Then the EDD (estimated delivery date) arrived. The midwife visited me with the interpreter and checked me over. She was touching my tummy to find where the baby's head was positioned in my womb and found no changes since the last appointment. She told me to go to the hospital for a scan. So I went to the hospital with the interpreter.

We met the consultant at the hospital who carried out the scan. He told me that it was impossible to have a natural birth. I was so disappointed when the doctor informed me that I must have a caesarean that I refused, as I wanted a natural birth.

I then contacted my partner and asked him to come to the hospital immediately as I was feeling uncomfortable and needed someone to talk to and to make a joint decision. The interpreter was with us from one o'clock that afternoon until seven in the evening. The consultant informed me that if I went home that night, it would be at my own risk as I would be ignoring the doctor's advice.

I couldn't take in all that the consultant had said. So after that, I decided to go home – I knew it was at my own risk. I realised that I couldn't stay at home forever and increase the risk to my baby and decided to return to the hospital the next morning. I was there for the next two weeks.

Then I was induced to start labour. Nothing happened for three days. Then on the fourth day, I started to have contractions and it got worse through the night. It was so painful. The consultant and the day staff arrived at nine o'clock in the morning. They looked at my birth plan, stating that I wanted to have a home birth and everything as natural as possible, which meant no pain relief. Because I was shaking, becoming weaker, they asked whether I wanted an epidural to relieve the pain I was going through. I thought to myself, what is the point of going on with all this pain when there is pain relief available to help me? So I reluctantly accepted an epidural and found it to be a nice relief, it made my body relax and I couldn't feel any pain. A nice feeling!

Then my midwife came into work. She had heard that I was in labour and came to support me all day. But her shift finished at six o'clock so she had to go. I was so disappointed to see her go as she was a brilliant support.

Then I had a different midwife. I had never met her before. I found it impossible to understand her because she had a strong accent and she found it difficult to understand me.* There was a lot of communication breakdown, especially when my contractions were so strong that I couldn't concentrate on what she was saying.

I had hired a birth stool from a specialist company for a month, really for my home birth. It works a bit like a toilet chair with a round seat and a hole in the middle and a bucket underneath to catch blood and amino fluids when the baby is born. The midwife couldn't work out how the stool worked. So instead, she told me to remain lying on the bed and keep pushing. I told her I wanted to use the birth stool. It suddenly became a battle with me trying to convince her what I wanted while I was in labour and about to give birth.

She reluctantly agreed and then put the stool on the bed. Clearly it wasn't safe. It was like having a chair on top of the bed – my partner had to hold the birth stool on the bed to stop me from falling off the stool and the bed. Both of us agreed that using the stool on the bed wasn't safe and told the midwife to put it on the floor.

I was in the second stage of labour from six o'clock right through the night until 3.30 in the morning, a total of nine and a half hours. The midwife said she could see my baby's head coming and encouraged me to keep pushing.

Then the consultant arrived. She had one look at me and told me that I needed to go to theatre for an assisted birth. The baby was in distress because both the baby and I were so tired and exhausted and that was affecting my baby's breathing. At the theatre, I was told that the consultant would be using forceps to bring my baby out. Then the consultant told me that my baby was too far back in my womb to use the forceps. I was so confused.

Then the consultant said that I would have to have an emergency caesarean immediately. It was no longer possible for me to have a natural birth. Then within five minutes, my daughter was brought out of my womb – I couldn't believe how quickly the caesarean was carried out and everything went blurred. I was sick from all the medication and epidurals and I hadn't had food for so many hours that I fell asleep with exhaustion.

I remember when the staff took my baby out and put her under the spotlight to check if she was OK. After five minutes, or so, they brought her close to my face but I couldn't cuddle her. I cried with joy and sadness at the same time.

I really wanted to complain to the hospital. I talked to several friends and relatives about my bitterness, they couldn't advise – it was wholly my decision. After time, having been joyful with my baby, the bitterness evaporated. I thought, well, we both made it, despite all medical intervention.

I couldn't wait to get home and get on with our lives and was looking forward to taking care of my baby, independently and confidently. We both recovered very quickly. Just looking at her face – her smile, her twinkly eyes, and asleep like an angel, you quickly forget the trauma of her birth.

*Lipreading someone with an unfamiliar accent can be difficult.

Maria's story

My first child was born without the use of painkillers since the student midwife was so encouraging and kept on saying, "you are doing brilliantly". Positive feedback did wonders for my body and I was thinking like this, "if I am doing brilliantly then I feel good about myself, then the pain is nothing and I can cope". She was just perfect, so easy to lipread and to talk to.

Because of the great first birth, I decided to have a home birth the second time. The midwives were fantastic and sat down to go through everything with me, all written down. They brought all the equipment required for the home birth – two big plastic boxes, full of interesting and strange instruments. I used to go into the spare room where the boxes were kept, touching them, trusting them and having a peek here and there.

But this home birth did not happen as I went almost a week and a bit over my due date. On the recommendation of the consultant, who took his time and explained everything very clearly about some build up of protein or something, I had to go into hospital to be induced.

This time around I had a male student midwife. He was very easy to lipread. Being induced took me by surprise as to how quickly my labour began and proceeded. There was a stage when my body's instincts started to push and the midwife was going "not yet, not yet" and there was no controlling my body. It was then he realised that my baby was in distress and swiftly got in senior staff to aid with the birth. My boy was born with the cord around his neck. If an interpreter had been there it wouldn't have worked as it was a very tense moment. The midwives worked quickly and my baby was fine after a short while – the student stayed for a bit then left us to drink in this magic moment alone, holding our baby.

I spent three days in the ward with my first child because she had developed a touch of jaundice. The midwives were kind in waking me up every couple of hours to feed her rather than myself relying on the alert pager which was hopeless.

After the birth of my second son I left on the day of giving birth so I didn't have to experience the sleepless nights again.

Sharon's story

My daughter was born at home – a planned home birth that was a very positive experience for the whole family. My son, then two years old, was able to sleep undisturbed – amazing considering the comings and goings of the midwives. It was really special being able to show him his two-hour-old sister when he woke up the next morning.

Throughout this labour I was very comfortable and could move around, eat and drink when I wanted to and giving birth was so much easier and quicker. I had lots of one-to-one attention from the midwives. Afterwards, they cleaned up everything – I could not find any traces of the birth, despite the mess – ran a bath and made me feel very supported.

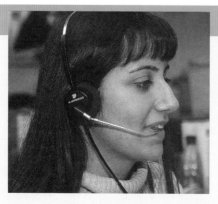

Further information

- Active Birth Centre
- www.babycentre.co.uk
- www.baby-parenting.co.uk
- www.babycaretens.co.uk
- Midwives Information and Resource Service
- National Childbirth Trust
- www.pulsar-tens.com

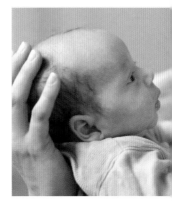

Chapter 11
Your baby's first few days

Checking your baby is healthy

First few hours

- As soon as your baby is born the midwife will give her a quick visual check and you probably won't even notice this being done. This is called the APGAR.
- Your baby will then be given a full 'top to toe' check, usually in the first hour after she has been born.

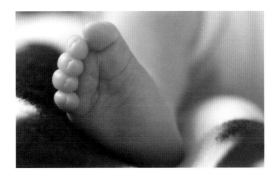

One or two days old

- A paediatrician – a doctor who specialises in the care of children – will give your baby a paediatric baby examination when she is one or two days old and before you take your baby home, if you have given birth in hospital. Some midwives are also qualified to do this examination. Midwives would always refer any baby to a paediatrician if there is any sign of a problem.
- If you have had a home birth your GP or specially qualified midwife can do the paediatric examination at home.

Care from your midwife – days one to 10

Home birth
After you have had your baby and delivered the placenta your midwife will check you and your baby. This will take at least one hour. She will then leave you to rest. You should have an adult staying with you. It could be your partner, mother, sister or friend. Perhaps one could stay during the day, and one at night.

- A midwife will come and visit you the next day, or if your baby is born early in the morning, later in the same day.

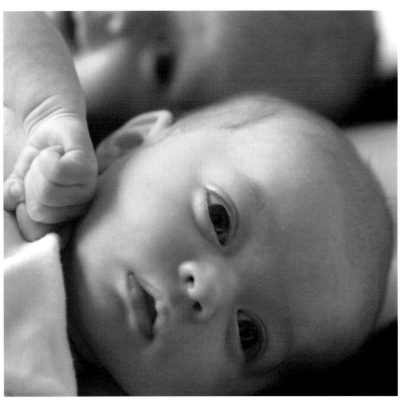

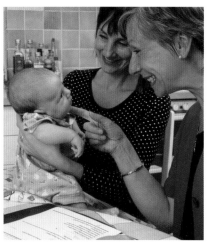

- They might then visit every day for a minimum of ten days, but the midwife will check if you need a visit every day.
  If you don't the midwife is more likely to visit about three times in the first ten days.
- They will tell you where you can find a drop-in clinic and give you a contact telephone number to call if you need help or advice. You will need to ask if there is a textphone or fax you can use. You will always be able to contact the maternity unit or hospital as well.

Hospital birth or GP unit

- If you have your baby in hospital, or in a GP unit, you will stay there between two to five days but if you have had a straightforward birth you may be able to go home after six hours.
- You will get the same level of care when you get back home as mothers who have given birth at home. You will be under the care of the community midwife for at least ten days.
- You may not see the same midwife each time but you are usually given written records and care plans to keep so you can show each midwife what has happened on earlier visits.

Julie's story

The midwives on the ward were brilliant to me, they helped me with my son as they looked after him during the night while I slept. The senior midwife arranged for me to use my mobile on the ward to contact my husband if I had any problems, or whatever. Normally they don't allow mobiles to be used in hospital but they made an exception for me.

Anja's story

The midwife came for a check up of the baby and me. I made sure that my hearing mother wasn't around then, because then the midwife would only talk to her, and not to me.

- The midwife will plan with you how often you need a visit. You will always be given a contact number. You will need to ask if there is a textphone or fax you can use. You can also always contact a midwife at the local maternity unit or hospital for advice.
- Your GP may also visit you at home, however, this varies across the country, so ask your GP before you have your baby.

What happens when the midwife visits?

Each time the midwife visits they:
- Will check how you are coping with the baby.
- May feel your abdomen to check that your womb is normal.
- Will ask about your 'vaginal loss' or 'lochia'– this is like a period (see *Chapter 16 Looking after yourself now you have a new baby* for more information).
- Will check that any stitches are healing.
- Will check that you are breastfeeding comfortably.
- May check your blood pressure.
- May check that you are eating and drinking healthily.
- May check that you are going to the toilet normally.
- Will check that you are doing your pelvic floor exercises.
- Will check that you are getting enough sleep and rest.
- Will check that you are feeling emotionally well.
- Will also check your baby.

You can discuss all this with your midwife before you have your baby, so that you know what to expect.

After 10 days

- Your midwife will advise you to make an appointment to visit your GP for a postnatal check when your baby is six weeks old. It is a good idea to book this as soon as you can.
- After 10 days, if everything is OK, the midwife will discharge you from their

care and the health visitor will take over. The midwife will make all these arrangements.

- If you had any problems when you were pregnant, or a caesarean section, you may be given a postnatal appointment to see the consultant obstetrician in the hospital. The hospital will usually send you details of the appointment or the midwife will arrange it for you.

Care from your health visitor

The health visitor will take over from the midwife after ten days. However, the midwife may still care for you for up to 28 days to give:

- Breastfeeding help.
- Help if your baby was in a special care baby unit and so did not go home until after ten days.
- Help if you have twins or triplets.
- Help if you feel physically or emotionally unwell.

The health visitor is usually based in the local health centre or GP surgery and will:

- Provide health screening, advice and education for families with babies and children.
- Run immunisation programmes for babies and young children.
- Run drop-in clinics for mothers with, for example, advice on feeding your baby.
- Visit new mothers at home, around ten days after your baby is born. However, this does not happen in all areas of the the country.

Your baby's umbilical cord

Minutes after your baby is born her umbilical cord will be cut to separate her from her placenta. She will be left with a short little cord attached to her tummy. The end will be clamped to stop any blood coming out of the cord. You should discuss cord cutting and clamping before your baby is born and put this in your birth plan. Sometimes you or your partner may wish to cut the cord. The midwife will usually take the clamp off between one and three days later.

Maria's story

My local health visitors are excellent. I had the same two health visitors for both children. I breastfed my daughter until she was 10 months and my son 11 months – both times the health visitors were encouraging.

I hardly used the alert system and only began to use it when they progressed into their 'big girl' or 'big boy' bedrooms. The health visitors commented on how alert and happy my children were as babies and toddlers and how they looked at me when I signed and talked to them, which was really rewarding.

Having children is special – the magic of seeing them laugh, smile and sign is just the beginning.

Looking after the cord

Your midwife will tell you how to look after the cord.

- You will probably be told to wipe the cord with clean water and to dry it with cotton wool once a day.
- Sometimes you will need to do it everytime you change your baby's nappy.
- Keep the nappy below the cord so the cord stays dry. The cord is often sticky but it will dry and shrivel up over the next few days.
- It will probably fall off when your baby is about ten days old.

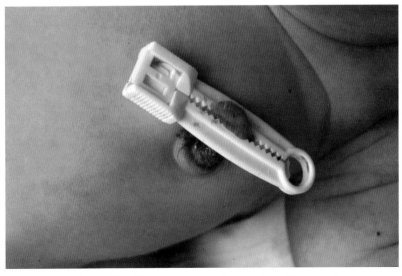

Your midwife will tell you how to look after the cord

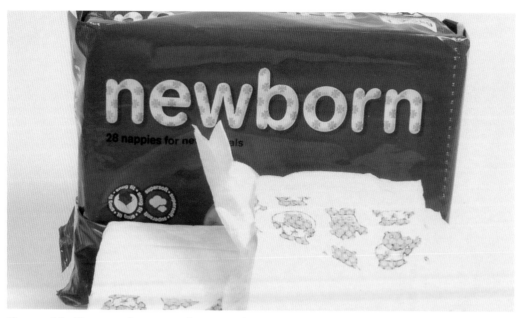

Your midwife can show you how to clean your baby and put on a nappy

Vitamin K

Many doctors recommend that all babies are given vitamin K when they are born. It is needed to help their blood clot. Your baby will develop vitamin K naturally once she has been feeding for a few days but for the first few days there is a risk that she could start bleeding anywhere in her body – vitamin K will help prevent this.

- Your baby can be given vitamin K by injection when she is checked by the midwife, after she has been born, *or*

- She can be given it in her mouth – but she will need to have several doses between her first day and when she is six weeks old.

When you are pregnant you can discuss this with your midwife or GP to help you decide what you want for your baby.

Nappies

Your baby won't wee a lot in her first few days. However, she will poo something called 'meconium'. This is a thick, greeny black and very sticky substance. As she starts to feed, the meconium will gradually become greenish-brown in colour. If you are breastfeeding and all is going well your baby's poo will start to be soft and bright yellow and smell quite nice. If you are bottle feeding, her poos will be more solid and pale yellowish brown and won't smell very nice!

How to put on a nappy

If you are having a hospital birth remember to take nappies with you. Your midwife can show you how to clean your baby and put on a nappy. You can use either disposable nappies or washable/reusable nappies (see *Chapter 3 Finding out you are pregnant* for more information).

Rosie's story

After the birth, I was moved into the postnatal ward. There were so many mothers in the ward, with their newborn babies. I started to feel isolated because the visiting hours were so short. My husband Sam had to go home. Communication with others in the ward was difficult. The television didn't have any subtitles. I saw other hearing mothers watching TV, listening to the radio, or chatting to each other. That left me annoyed and irritated. I had no choice but to read magazines and wait for visiting hours before my husband or my mother came.

Also, during the first night after my baby was born, I was asleep and I couldn't hear my baby crying. The baby alarm that vibrates wouldn't work as the ward had many crying babies and the alarm kept going off. So I told the nurse to alert me if my baby cried while I was sleeping, but she didn't. Instead, she woke me and had a go at me, saying "your daughter has been crying". I told her that I couldn't hear my daughter crying so how could I know if she had been crying?

Jaundice

What is jaundice?

When you are pregnant your baby gets oxygen from you. This is passed to her through the placenta and umbilical cord. Babies' blood contains extra red blood cells to move oxygen around the body. Once babies are born and breathing through their own lungs, they no longer need the extra red blood cells and their body will begin to get rid of them.

These extra red blood cells are broken down in your baby's spleen. This creates a by-product called bilirubin. Your baby's liver should help get rid of her bilirubin. However, because her liver is not very developed, she may not be able to cope with the bilirubin in the first days of life. Too much bilirubin in the bloodstream will make your baby's skin look yellow or jaundiced.

A small amount of jaundice is quite normal. However, if there is too much bilirubin in your baby's blood, it could affect her brain. Your midwife and doctor will carefully check any jaundice in your baby and tell you how you can help her.

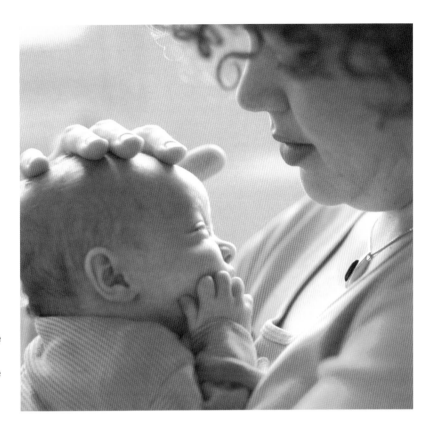

How is jaundice treated?

If your baby becomes very jaundiced, she will be placed under a mobile phototherapy unit which gives out light. The light is pleasantly warm and will not hurt. The midwives or nurses will do special checks – such as keeping your baby's eyes protected from the light with a blindfold.

Jaundice doesn't usually last for a long time. Your baby may need only a few hours' treatment, or possibly a couple of days. She can usually be treated at your bedside so there is no need for you to be separated.

Patricia's story

My daughter was in intensive care. She did her first poo (meconium) in the womb just before she came out. The poo was a green and sticky fluid and poisonous and the baby swallowed a bit which is dangerous. As a result of this, she had a lung infection and had to have antibiotics via a drip to treat the infection for a week. It was so awful to see her like this, her tiny hand was bandaged around the needle and every two days, the needle had to be reinserted into her other hand. The needle looked too big for her tiny hand and if she bent her hand, it would have been really painful, hence the bandage from her hand all the way up to her wrist/lower arm. My daughter also had jaundice but that was easy to treat and disappeared after a few days.

Farah's story

There was excitement at the hospital and I had numerous visitors, both staff and public, wanting to see my baby.* I was so tired and was not expecting those visitors. They didn't explain why they were there in my room. I had my own room separate from the ward as I felt I didn't want to face any communication problems that may arise if I was on the ward. I was more comfortable in my own room, spending time with my baby, apart from the constant interruption from the many visitors who couldn't believe how big my baby was.

*Farah had a big baby, see *Chapter 10 Labour and birth*.

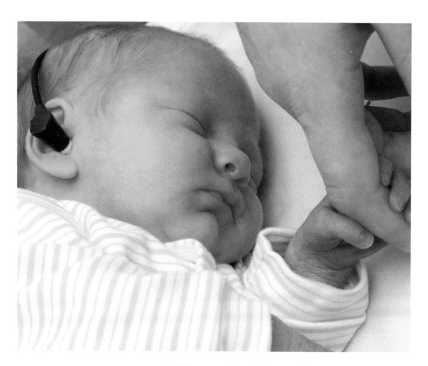

What is Newborn Hearing Screening?

Newborn Hearing Screening is the screening of newborn babies to see if they are deaf, within the first few hours or days of life. It used to be known as Universal Neonatal Hearing Screening (UNHS).

Newborn Hearing Screening is being introduced across the UK in stages. It may already be available in your area. If it is, your baby will be screened in her first few weeks. If you have had a hospital birth this may be done before you leave hospital or it may be carried out at home, or in your local surgery or health clinic. Your midwife will give you more information about your baby's screening test.

It is becoming routine for all babies to be screened to see if they are deaf. If you live in a Newborn Hearing Screening area you will be asked for your consent before your baby is screened. If you have any concerns about the screening process discuss them with your midwife.

Contact the RNID Information Line to find out if Newborn Hearing Screening is available in your area.

You can also get a range of information from The National Deaf Children's Society and the Newborn Hearing Screening Programme. This includes leaflets that

Tips for your stay in hospital

- Make sure you visit the hospital before the birth and talk to the staff about your communication needs.
- Ask the staff to label your chart/file 'D/deaf mother', or use your own way of letting staff know you are D/deaf.
- You may be able to ask for a private room if you prefer.
- Many maternity wards have an intercom system for security reasons. You will need to ask staff to make alternative arrangements to let you or your partner into the ward.
- You will not be able to use a mobile phone in hospital unless you go outside. Let staff know that you will need access to a textphone, or fax machine.
- If there is a television ask them to make sure you can view subtitles on it. See *Chapter 19 Your rights under the Disability Discrimination Act (1995)* for more information.
- You can get baby monitors for deaf parents. See *Chapter 3 Finding out you are pregnant.* Your baby monitor may go off every time a baby cries, not just your own, so ask the staff to let you know if they hear your baby crying.
- Give your baby lots of cuddles – she will enjoy being cuddled a lot and you will be able to see when she is ready to be fed by the movement of her mouth, without waiting for her to cry.

Julie's story

My mother came with me when we took my son to the hospital for his hearing test. The audiologist was very helpful, she made sure that I got the full information, by explaining how the process works. Then she carried out the test and confirmed that my son is hearing. I was pleased to know that my son is hearing after all as I know I don't need to worry about his future.

explain every stage of Newborn Hearing Screening. You will be given these leaflets if you live in an area where Newborn Hearing Screening has been introduced. You can also get a signed and subtitled video all about screening. Ask your midwife for a copy before you have your baby so you know what to expect.

What is targeted Newborn Hearing Screening?

In many areas hospitals already screen some babies if they are known to be at a higher risk of being deaf, for example, if your family has a history of deafness or if your baby has been in a Special Care Baby Unit for more than 48 hours. This kind of testing is called Targeted Newborn Hearing Screening.

Targeted screening aims to find out if your baby is deaf, as early as possible. By the end of 2005 all babies will be routinely screened for deafness. If you are not happy, remember you can say "no".

Katie's story

As my deafness is understood to be genetic, I was aware my baby might inherit this. The Newborn Hearing Screening was done when my baby was a day old. I had wondered whether to wait six weeks but was curious to find out. The staff were professional and explained what they were doing. The results were positive, although our baby's hearing loss may develop later.

Anja's story

When my son was three weeks old, we went for a Neonatal Hearing Screening for him. I did not know if he could hear, so I was happy to have the test so quickly. When it showed that he was hearing, I had quite mixed feelings. On the one hand I was happy for him to be hearing, on the other hand, perhaps selfishly, I quite liked the idea of another deaf person in the family.

What does Newborn Hearing Screening involve?

Newborn Hearing Screening is not painful or unpleasant for your child in any way. It can even be done as your baby sleeps. The person carrying out the test inserts a tiny probe just inside your baby's ear. The probe makes a small sound. If your baby's cochlea, or inner ear, responds normally, it produces a kind of 'echo' in response to the sound, and the probe picks this up. Both ears are checked.

If your baby's ear does not produce an 'echo', it does not mean that your baby is deaf – just that more tests are needed to find out whether you child's ear responds, or not.

Will I be offered support if my baby is deaf?

If your baby is deaf, this will not normally be confirmed until she is two to three months old, after she has had other tests to follow up the first screening. If she is deaf there are a range of choices and services available to you as a family. These depend on the level of your baby's deafness and the way you think about these may change over time. Whatever you decide to do in the long term, it is important to know that you will be able to get support from a range of agencies from the time that your child is identified as deaf.

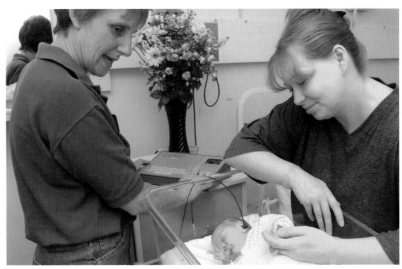

Newborn Hearing Screening is not painful or unpleaseant for your baby

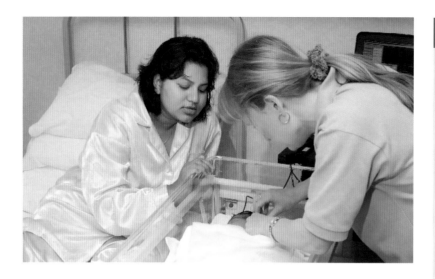

The Guthrie test

- All babies are given the Guthrie test when they are five to seven days old but only if you give permission. The test is to detect metabolic disorders that can be treated by giving your baby special milk or medicine.
- The test involves pricking your baby's heel to get several spots of blood. The test is easier if your baby's heel is warm. Put a sock on her heel several hours before the test.
- The test results usually take up to four weeks so the midwife has usually stopped visiting you by this time. The health visitor will let you know if the test has to be repeated or if there are any problems.

Discuss the Guthrie test with your midwife before you have your baby, so you know what to expect.

Patricia's story

On the fourth day after my baby was born a person from the Newborn Hearing Screening came to test my baby. She carried out the test but it wasn't clear. She thought it was maybe that my baby's ear was blocked with fluid from the birth and hadn't been cleaned since. I think she suspected that my baby might be deaf but she never told me.

She had been asking me lots of questions about my family history especially about my deaf parents and deaf brother. It didn't occur to me how important that information was for her. So I answered her questions where possible and thought she was asking too many questions and maybe invading my privacy. Then six weeks later, it was confirmed that my baby is deaf.

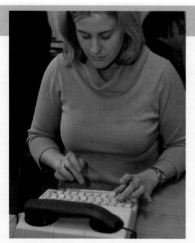

Further information

- www.deafnessatbirth.org.uk
- National Childbirth Trust
- National Deaf Children's Society
- Newborn Hearing Screening Programme www.nhsp.info
- RNID Information Line

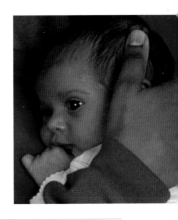

Chapter 12
Feeding your baby

It's up to you whether you breastfeed or bottle feed your baby but have a look at why breastfeeding is good for you and your baby before making that decision.

Breastfeeding

Why is breastmilk good for my baby?

- Breastmilk contains antibodies – these help to protect your baby from infections. Bottle fed babies are much more likely to get severe infections such as gastroenteritis, which may mean your baby needs to go to hospital.
- Your baby will have a lower risk of diabetes.
- Your baby will have less chance of getting eczema (a skin condition that can make your baby's skin dry, hot and itchy and occasionally bleed).
- Your baby will be more mentally alert and active.
- Your baby's nappies will be less smelly.

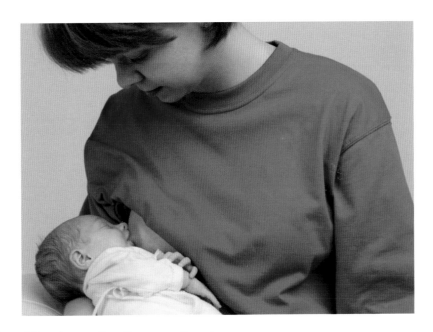

After six months, if you continue to breastfeed while your baby starts to eat other foods, this will still be good for both of you. You can carry on breastfeeding for as long as you and your baby are happy.

How long should I breastfeed for?

Your baby will benefit most from having only breastmilk for around the first six months of her life. She will get all the food and drink she needs and have some protection against a range of illnesses.

Is breastfeeding better for me?

- The longer you breastfeed over your lifetime the lower your risk of getting breast cancer.
- You will have stronger bones in later life.
- Your body will get back to a similar shape to the one it was before you had your baby, more quickly.

Patricia's story

My baby was in a special baby care unit after a complicated birth. I was determined that I was going to breastfeed her. The staff said fine. When she was hungry they would phone my ward staff to let me know when to go down and breastfeed her. This meant about every two hours, the staff alerted me to go and see my baby, even during the night. I also bought a flashing light portable system. The ward staff had a transmitter and alerted me whenever my baby needed me. I can't remember exactly how it works, but it works!

I went down to the special care unit to breastfeed my baby. I found breastfeeding easy. I was lucky that my baby latched on quite quickly without any problem. I was told that there was a breastfeeding counsellor in the special care unit. The first time I breastfed I was trying to find the best way to hold my baby and to encourage her to latch on, then the counsellor came over. She was a mother herself. She corrected me by explaining and demonstrating to me.

Anyway, I breastfed easily without any problems. When my baby was better and was moved into my ward I breastfed her from my bed and bonded well with her. I remember looking at her while breastfeeding and thinking to myself, "wow, my baby!".

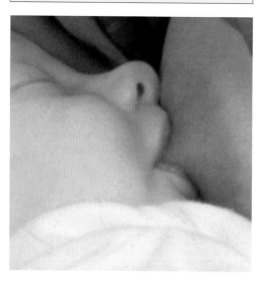

How will I know how to breastfeed?

Your midwife or other hospital staff, such as a healthcare support worker, should show you how to breastfeed soon after you have given birth. Ask them to guide you again if you want more help, until you have learned to do it yourself.

Tips for breastfeeding

- You don't need any special preparation for breastfeeding but it's a good idea to look after yourself by eating a healthy diet.
- Sit in an upright chair, or use pillows or cushions to support you and your baby.
- Make sure your knees aren't sloping down. You can support your feet on a stool or pile of telephone directories.
- Try to make sure your baby is calm before you start.
- Turn your baby towards you and keep her back and head in a straight line. Make sure your baby's nose is in line with your nipple.
- Make sure she can move her head so that she can tilt it back as she comes onto your breast.
- Touch your baby's mouth with your nipple. Wait a few moments till she opens her mouth really wide. Then move her gently but firmly on to the end of your breast. Your nipple and probably most of the darker skin around your nipple (the areola) will be in her mouth. Her chin should be firmly against your breast.
- Let your baby finish the first breast before offering her the second.
- If you need to stop her sucking, don't pull her away. Instead, put your little finger gently in the side of her mouth to break the suction. Your midwife will show you how.
- Don't worry if you don't get it right first time, you may need to try several times.
- If you give your baby bottles as well as breastfeeding her in the early days it can interfere with breastfeeding.

How will I know if I've got it right?

- Breastfeeding should not hurt you (see later for more information).
- Your breasts should also feel comfortable.
- You may feel an unusual deep feeling in your breast as your baby draws your milk out of you.
- Your baby's mouth will be wide open.
- She should be suckling you, that means her tongue should be squeezing out the milk, rather than sucking on your nipple.
- You should be able to see her lower jaw moving up and down.
- She will stop when she has had enough milk.

How often should I breastfeed?

You should breastfeed your baby when she is hungry. You will learn to recognise the signs that she wants feeding, long before she starts crying. Look out for her stretching her body and opening her mouth. How often she wants to feed may vary a lot. Most young babies need at least eight feeds in every 24-hour period. She will usually feed for around 20 to 40 minutes at first. The feeds will get shorter as she grows and feeds more strongly.

Can I breastfeed if I have had a caesarean?

Yes. You can breastfeed if you have had a caesarean but you may find you need more help to begin with. Get advice and tips from your midwife or health visitor.

What if breastfeeding hurts?

Breastfeeding should *not* hurt. If it does ask your midwife or health visitor for help. You can also get information and support from the National Childbirth Trust and other breastfeeding support organisations (see *Chapter 21 Further information* for contact details).

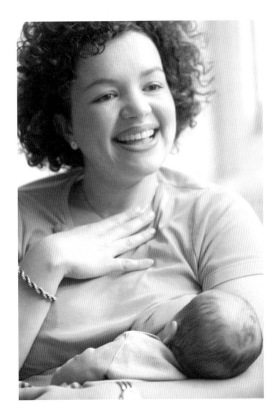

I'm finding breastfeeding really difficult, what should I do?

Speak to your midwife or health visitor and contact the National Childbirth Trust or other support organisations for information and support (see *Chapter 21 Further information* for contact details).

What if my baby won't breastfeed?

You can squeeze milk from your breasts – known as 'expressing' – by hand, or by using a breast pump. A midwife or breastfeeding counsellor can show you how to give your expressed milk to your baby using a small cup – known as 'cup feeding'.

Jennifer's story

With breastfeeding, I was really lucky because a National Childbirth Trust breastfeeding counsellor visited my ward when I had my eldest. At that time I was a bit depressed and wasn't happy with the way I breastfed. She had the right attitude and was very patient with me with communication. She drew diagrams and wrote down if I didn't understand. I didn't have any problems with breastfeeding afterwards.

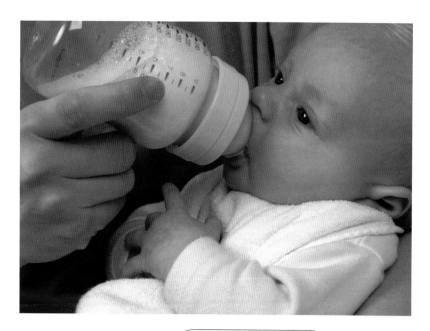

Bottle feeding

Ask your midwife or heath visitor to show you how to bottle feed. If you choose to bottle feed, you need to know that it is expensive. You need to buy bottles, teats, formula milk and a way of sterilising the equipment.

If you give birth in hospital you may need to take the bottle feeding equipment and baby milk in with you. Check with your midwife.

What will I need for bottle feeding?

- Powdered milk or ready-made milks suitable for newborn babies. This is often known as formula milk. Ask your midwife or health visitor to advise which type of formula milk to buy for your baby. You will need to add the powder to freshly boiled water. You should follow the instructions on the container when making it. It is important to get the mix right or you might make your baby ill.
- A kettle.
- At least six 250ml feeding bottles. You need these to put the milk in.
- A bottle brush to clean the bottles.
- A steriliser or some other way of sterilising bottles. **It is very important that you keep your baby's bottles and teats and other equipment used in bottle feeding very clean by sterilising them. If you do not, your baby can be ill.** Ask your midwife or health visitor to show you how to sterilise everything. You can also get leaflets with pictures from some of the organisations listed at the end of this chapter.
- The 'teats' are the rubbery bits that go on the end of the bottles and in your baby's mouth. You can get special teats for newborn babies. You should not use any teats that are cracked or sticky.
- A soft brush to clean the teats.
- A large, wide-based jug for hot water. You can use this to re-heat bottles.

Anja's story

I didn't really think about breastfeeding or bottle feeding. I just decided to breastfeed. It was not really easy at the beginning, because both the baby and I had to learn how to do it, and it was also quite painful, with bleeding from my nipples, but I just carried on, and after two or three weeks it was so easy to do, and I could always express milk if I wanted to go somewhere without the baby. I breastfed until I had to go back to work. Then I started to bottle feed the baby, and I thought that breastfeeding was so much easier.

I thought that breastfeeding my other children would be very easy, because I had experience, and the second one was indeed easy, but the third one was quite difficult, and I nearly had breast inflammation (mastitis), which was not very nice! I was told it was only a problem with positioning. I thought – I have had two children before, and they were positioned in the same way, and I never had problems like this! It turned out that the baby had thrush, but only after I read something about it in a magazine. I thought – that looks like what I have got and I asked the doctor about it. She gave me medicine. Now I am still breastfeeding her at five months old. When I am at work, my husband gives her formula.

Milk tokens

If you are on benefits you are entitled to milk tokens. You can exchange these for seven pints of milk a week, this is for you to drink if you are breastfeeding. This may change so you will need to check – contact the Maternity Alliance (see *Chapter 21 Further information*).

- A fridge to store the milk in. You can make up a whole day's bottles and keep them in the fridge but throw away any milk you have not used after 24 hours.
- If you are on benefits you are entitled to milk tokens which you can exchange for 900g of formula a week. This may change so you will need to check – contact the Maternity Alliance for information (see *Chapter 21 Further information*).

Tips for bottle feeding

- Calm your baby before you start feeding her.
- Make sure your chair has good back support and use pillows to help you support your baby.
- Make sure your knees don't slope towards the floor.
- Practise different ways to hold your baby until you find the one she likes best, but keep her head higher than her tummy.
- Check the milk is the correct temperature by testing a bit on the inside of your arm. It should not be too hot. Do not use a microwave to heat any baby milk. You may burn your baby's mouth.
- Put the teat of the bottle gently against your baby's mouth and wait for her to open her mouth.
- Hold the bottle in the same way you hold a pencil. Try to keep the teat full of milk to stop her sucking in air.
- Bottle feeding is hard work so your baby will stop for rests.
- If she gasps, stop feeding and sit her upright.

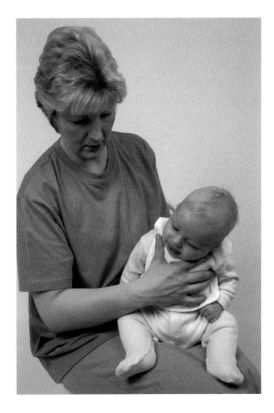

- If the teat looks flat take it out so that air can get back in it again.
- When she stops sucking, gently take the teat from her mouth. Don't try to force her to empty the bottle.
- Sit her upright or rest her against your shoulder. Rub her back gently. She may burp but not always. This is known as 'winding'.
- It's OK to give her more milk from the bottle she has just been sucking from but only for the next 10 minutes. If she wants more milk after 10 minutes you must start again with new milk.

Cleaning the bottle and teat after you have used them

- Afterwards, rinse the bottle and teat in cold water.
- Then wash them both in warm soapy water using a bottle brush to check the bottle is clean.
- Then rinse in clear water.
- Finally, sterilise the bottle and teat again.

You should also...

sterilise dummies, bowls, spoons, breast pumps and teethers.

How much milk should I bottle feed my baby?

Your baby won't need a lot of milk in her first few days but she will get hungrier as she gets bigger. Feed her whenever she lets you know she is hungry. She won't always want the same amount of milk. She will let you know when she has had enough so don't force her.

I'm finding bottle feeding difficult, what should I do?

Ask your midwife or health visitor for advice.

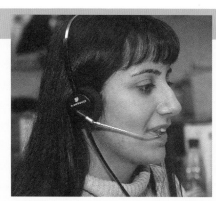

Further information

- Ask your midwife or health visitor if you need any more information about feeding your baby. They can also give you the telephone numbers of your local trained breastfeeding counsellors.
- Association of Breastfeeding Mothers
- www.breastfeeding.co.uk
- The Breastfeeding Network
- Department of Health publications (see *Useful reading* in *Chapter 21 Further information*).
- La Leche League
- Maternity Alliance
- Midwives Information and Resource Service
- National Childbirth Trust including their Breastfeeding line
- The UNICEF UK Baby Friendly Initiative

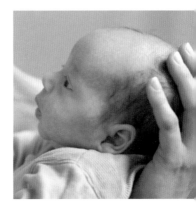

Chapter 13
Premature babies

What does 'premature baby' mean?

A premature baby is born too early – before the 37th week of pregnancy. Today, more and more premature babies survive, but unfortunately some premature babies still die because their bodies are so fragile.

Why are some babies born prematurely?

Some women start labour prematurely – that is before their baby is due to be born. Researchers don't always know why this happens, however, the main causes are:

- If you are having more than one baby at the same time, for example, twins, triplets or quads. This is known as a 'multiple pregnancy'.
- If the neck of your womb is weak.
- If your womb is an unusual shape.
- If you have an infection.
- If you smoke.
- If you use some illegal drugs.

If you have already had one or more premature babies, your chances of having another premature baby are higher.

Can anything be done to try and stop premature labour?

If you go into labour and you are less than about 32 weeks pregnant your doctor may use drugs to try to stop the labour. This is so that you can be given an injection of steroids to help the baby's lungs to mature and develop. This can help prevent respiratory distress syndrome (see below). The drugs used to stop labour are often effective for 24 hours or more, which is enough time for the steroids to work. They may make your heart rate go up.

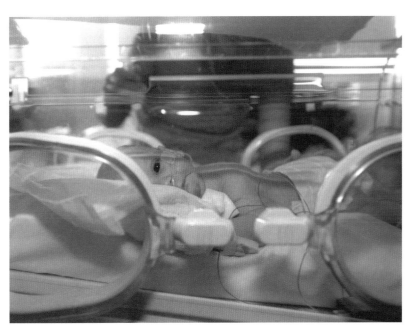

All premature babies spend some time in a special care baby unit

Sometimes doctors may decide to deliver a baby early to try to save the baby's life and/or that of the mother. The main reasons for this are if the mother has:

- Pre-eclampsia. We tell you more about this in *Chapter 8 If things go wrong during pregnancy.*

- A urinary tract (where your wee comes out) infection, or other infection.
- Diabetes. We tell you more about this in *Chapter 8 If things go wrong during pregnancy.*
- Placenta praevia. This is when the placenta is covering the cervix. It means the placenta is in front of the baby's head. If the cervix starts to open a bit it may be a risk for the baby.
- Placental abruption. This is when the placenta separates from the womb.
- Your baby may also be delivered early if she is not growing properly or has foetal distress. This means your baby is showing signs that something is not right, such as a slow heart beat.

What happens when a baby is born prematurely?

If a baby is born prematurely she won't be as strong as other babies. She could have a range of problems. These include:

- **Respiratory distress syndrome (RDS)**
  This is the term used to describe breathing problems in newborn babies and, especially, premature babies. Your baby may need artificial ventilation to help her breathe.
- **Bronchopulmonary dysplasia**
  If a baby has been on a ventilator for a long time or has had treatment with oxygen for a long time the lungs don't develop properly. The medical term for this is dysplasia. This means that the lungs don't work so well. The baby's heart then has to work harder to pump oxygen round the body and may fail.
- **Intraventricular haemorrhage**
  Premature babies, especially those born before 33 weeks, are particularly at risk from bleeding from the fragile blood vessels in the brain. In a very few cases this can cause severe brain damage and may lead to a condition known as hydrocephalus – water on the brain. While some babies may be severely affected, others get over it relatively easily.

- **Infections**
  Premature babies are particularly at risk from infections. They might get these from the womb or whilst they are being born. Unfortunately they do not have the ability to fight infections as well as babies born later in pregnancy.

How are premature babies cared for?

All premature babies spend some time in a special care baby unit. These are also known as neonatal units. Some babies may need to be transferred to an intensive care unit at a different hospital where there are specially trained staff and special facilities. Premature babies are cared for 24 hours a day by staff who have a wide range of technology to help them.

If your baby is premature she will be put in an incubator, which looks like a small cabinet. You can see your baby through the sides of the incubator. The incubator will keep your baby supplied with warmth, air and oxygen to help her breathe. A door in the top of the incubator allows you and the nurses to reach in to look after your baby.

Your baby will have sticky patches placed on her skin, and wires from these will link her to monitors. These will be used to check her breathing, heart rate and temperature.

Can I give my baby breastmilk?

Until your baby is strong enough to breastfeed or take a bottle, she will be fed and given drugs via tiny tubes. If you want to you may be able to express breast milk to feed your baby. The nurses in the special care baby unit and/or the midwives on the ward will help you.

Breastmilk is particularly good for premature babies. Some hospitals have a 'milk bank'. This provides pasteurised breastmilk, donated by other mothers, for premature babies whose mothers can't provide expressed milk for them.

Your feelings when you have a premature baby

If your baby is premature, instead of feeling excited you are likely to feel very worried and distressed. Premature babies have a difficult start but the majority do well. However, it can be upsetting if your baby is in an incubator so that you cannot hold her in your arms or breastfeed her straightaway, as you had hoped. The staff on the special care baby unit will help you to learn to make contact with your baby and to bond with her.

How much time should I spend with my baby?

Premature babies still need the same love and attention as full-term babies. Try to spend as much time as possible with your baby. At first, you will probably be in the hospital with your baby. Once you have returned home it is important to visit the hospital often and stay as long as you can.

Usually mums and dads can visit whenever they like. Sometimes other relatives can visit but staff do prefer to keep visitors to a minimum in order to prevent your baby getting an infection.

Will I be able to touch my baby?

You will be encouraged to touch and stroke your baby when she is in the incubator. When your baby is well enough to come out of the incubator the staff will support you and encourage you to hold your baby. Cuddling and stroking your baby will help her grow and thrive.

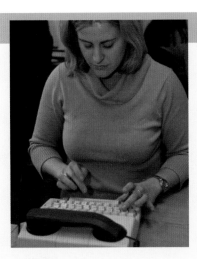

Further information

- BLISS
- National Childbirth Trust
- WellBeing

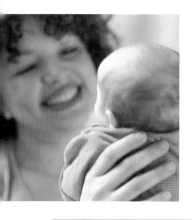

Chapter 14
Your baby's first few weeks at home

Although our book is mainly written for deaf women who are pregnant, or planning to get pregnant, we thought it would be useful to include some general information to help you through the first few weeks at home with your baby. This is only a brief look at some of the common things new mums want to know about. We also give you details of where you can go for more information.

Registering your baby's birth

- You must register your baby within six weeks of her being born.
- Some hospitals offer a registration service whilst you are staying on the maternity ward but if they don't you will need to go to your nearest registry office. Most hospitals will be able to give you the address but you will find them listed in your telephone book under your 'local authority'. If you live in Northern Ireland they will be listed under 'Registration of births, deaths and marriages'.
- If you are married to your baby's father, you, or your husband, can register your baby.
- If you are not married you have to go yourself. If you are not married and want the father's name to go on the birth certificate he must go with you to the registry office.

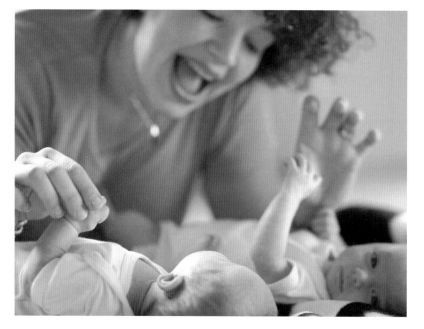

Keeping your baby clean

New babies don't get very dirty and don't need to be bathed every day. In fact many don't like being bathed at all! All you really need to wash your baby is warm water and towels, with some cooled boiled water and cotton wool for washing her face. However, many parents choose to bath their baby in a baby bath, but you could use a large washing-up bowl or the

How to 'top and tail' your baby

You will need:

- **Clean warm water in two small bowls, or a special top and tail container.**

- **Two small flannels or cotton wool.**

- **A towel to lay your baby on.**

➤ Wash your hands before washing your baby.

➤ Using water from the first bowl of water, wash each of your baby's eyes with a separate piece of cotton wool, stroking gently away from her nose. The midwife may suggest you use water that you have boiled and allowed to cool, if your baby's eyes are sticky.

➤ Using clean cotton wool, gently clean her face and neck with particular attention to folds of skin and behind her ears.

➤ Pat her dry.

➤ Using clean cotton wool, clean her bottom using water from the second bowl of water. If you use plenty of water you can be gentle. Again pay special attention to folds of skin.

➤ Always wipe from front to back.

➤ If you have a baby boy, do not try to pull the skin back at the top of his penis.

➤ Baby boys often choose to wee at this time, so you can hold a flannel or piece of cotton wool over his penis.

➤ Pat your baby dry.

➤ You may want to tell your baby what you are doing. Keep eye contact and smile at her.

➤ Roll her onto her side to clean her back, rather than pulling her up on to her upper back and neck.

➤ When you have finished, wash your hands.

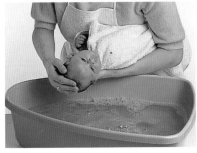
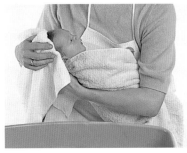
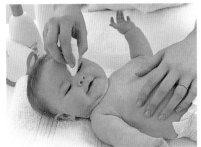
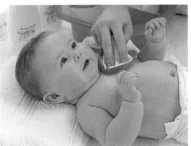
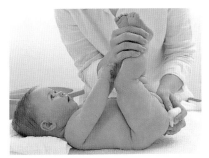
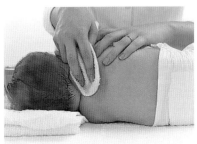
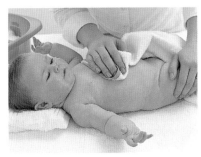

sink (watch out for the hot tap and wrap a flannel round it).

You might like to also buy:
- A bath thermometer.
- A baby sponge.
- A 'baby bather' or bath rest made of stretch fabric or sponge.

Should I keep my baby out of the sun?

Yes. Babies and small children need special care to protect them from the sun. The sun can very easily damage their skin and even mild sunburn is painful for a baby.

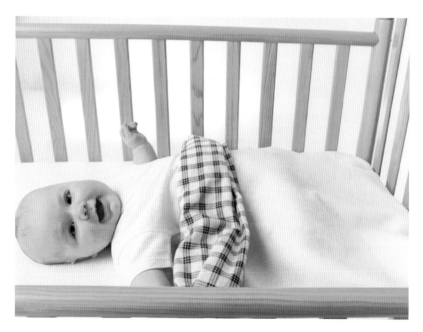

To reduce the risk of 'cot death' place your baby with her feet at the bottom of the cot

What is cot death or Sudden Infant Death Syndrome (SIDS)?

If a baby dies suddenly and there doesn't appear to be any obvious reason why she has died then this may be described as a 'cot death'.

Is there anything I can do to reduce the risk of cot death?

Yes. An organisation called The Foundation for the Study of Infant Deaths recommends you follow these key steps:

- Cut smoking in pregnancy – fathers too.
- Do not let anyone smoke in the same room as your baby.
- Place your baby on her back to sleep.
- Do not let your baby get too hot.
- Don't cover your baby's head – place her with her feet at the bottom of the cot, to stop her wriggling down under the covers.
- It is safest to sleep your baby in a cot in your bedroom for the first six months.
- Do not share a bed with your baby if you or your partner:
  - Are smokers (no matter where or when you smoke).
  - Have been drinking alcohol.
  - Take drugs or medication that make you drowsy.
  - Feel very tired.
- Do not sleep on a sofa, armchair or settee with your baby.

If your baby is unwell, get medical advice quickly.

To protect your baby:
- Cover your baby up. Use light-cotton, long-sleeved t-shirts and trousers.
- Keep babies and children out of the sun, especially in the middle of the day when it is strongest. They also need protection from the wind.
- Use a sun cream that is labelled at least factor 25, or a complete sun block.
- Get your baby a broad-brimmed sun hat. Use the shade on your pram or buy clip-on sunshades or a parasol to keep the sun off your baby.
- Check you have covered her feet.
- Put a window shade in your car.
- You can treat your baby's sunburn with cool baths and calamine lotion but if she gets burnt and her skin is blistered ask your GP for advice. **If you are at all concerned about your baby's sunburn contact your GP.**

Anja's story

My first two children used to go to a nursery. They enjoyed it very much, but I was not sure if I wanted the same for my third child. So when my eldest child started school, I met a deaf mum whose children were at the same school, and she was a registered childminder, and what was more, she had a vacant place coming up. Now my two youngest children are going to her, and they both love it. I have no issues about communication with her, and for the children it is quite normal.

Get medical help quickly

Check with your GP or health visitor about how to contact them out-of-hours. It may be easiest to take your baby to a hospital casualty department (A&E) if you are worried.

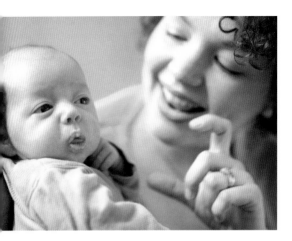

Playing with your baby

It is important to learn to play and communicate with your baby. In the first few days and weeks you are new to each other. If you watch your baby you can learn a lot about what makes her feel happy and safe and how to improve your communication with her. She probably won't smile until she is six weeks old but you can still learn what makes her feel happy before that.

Try to find time every morning and afternoon to play with your baby – 10 minutes is fine. Find out what she is watching and talk to her. Touch is also important. You might want to count her fingers and toes, stroke her tummy or hold her and dance. The better you and your baby know and understand each other, the more confident you will feel and the more you will enjoy being her mum.

Thinking about your baby's next few months

- As your baby grows and develops over the next few months you will need to start thinking about immunisation – getting your baby vaccinated against diseases. Your baby should have her first vaccination at two months. Ask your health visitor, midwife or GP for more information.
- If you need any advice or information over the next few months speak to your GP or health visitor or contact one of the organisations listed in *Chapter 21 Further information*.

Where can I find out about childcare?

For more information about finding childcare contact the Daycare Trust. Nurseries and childminders often have long waiting lists so start looking as early as you can – as soon as you are pregnant.

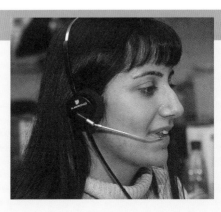

Further information

- www.babycentre.co.uk
- Child Accident Prevention Trust
- Daycare Trust
- Foundation for the Study of Infant Deaths
- www.immunisation.org.uk
- National Childbirth Trust
- National Deaf Children's Society
- RNID Information Line
- UNICEF UK Baby Friendly Initiative

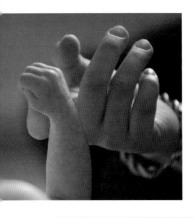

Chapter 15
What to do if you are worried about your baby

In this section we have included some basic information about common illnesses that your baby may have. **Do not just rely on the information we have given in this book. You should always seek proper medical help if you are at all concerned about your baby.**

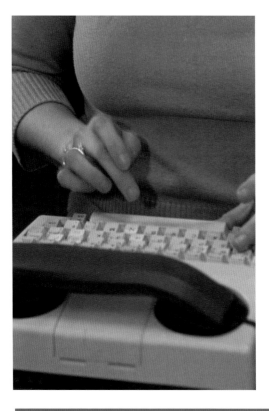

The following are signs that your baby may be ill

- She is not feeding normally.
- She has been sick a lot.
- She is breathing very quickly.
- She has had fewer than four wet nappies in the last 24 hours.
- She is irritable.
- There is blood in her poo or wee.
- She won't stop crying or her crying sounds different.
- She has no energy or she's floppy.
- She has a skin rash.
- She is very hot to touch, or very cold or clammy.
- She is very pale, or her skin is a different colour from normal.

Remember, always call your GP or health visitor if you are worried.

Who should I contact if I am worried about my baby?

- **If you are worried about your baby call your GP or health visitor.**
- **You can also contact NHS Direct for general health advice.**
- **Textphone users: 0845 606 4647 or 18001 0845 606 4647.**
- **Voice telephone users: 0845 4647.**

Call an ambulance if your baby

- Stops breathing, or goes blue.
- Does not respond and does not seem to be aware of what is going on.
- Has glazed eyes and does not focus on anything.
- Cannot be woken.
- Has a seizure (fit). Even if your baby recovers on her own, still call your GP.

To call an ambulance

- **Textphone users: Dial 18000. This is the number for BT TextDirect Emergency Services. You do not need to dial 999. Dialling 18000 on its own gives you a direct connection to the emergency services.**
- **Voice telephone users: Dial 999.**

Nappy rash

If your baby's bottom is very sore and red then she may have a nappy rash. You can help your baby by:
- Changing her nappy often, especially after a poo.
- Drying her bottom thoroughly after changing her nappy, or leaving her without a nappy to let her bottom dry.
- Using warm water and cotton wool instead of soap or babywipes.
- Applying a cream, such as zinc and castor oil cream.
- Washing reusable/washable nappies in non-biological washing powder and rinsing them very thoroughly.

If you are worried about your baby's nappy rash ask your GP or midwife for advice.

Thrush

If your baby's nappy rash seems to be very bad or won't get better she may have thrush. Visit your GP as this is an infection that needs to be treated by your GP.

A temperature

Taking your baby's temperature
The only really accurate way of taking your baby's temperature is by using an ear thermometer. These are quite expensive and you don't really need one. Instead you can test your baby's 'core temperature' by placing your hand flat on the skin of her chest or back. If your baby feels just warm, she's fine. If she feels hot, cold or clammy call your GP for advice. It is normal for your baby's hands and feet to feel cold.

Meningitis

Meningitis is extremely rare. The symptoms usually include a fever and your baby will not seem well. She might also:
- Be sick (vomit).
- Have a stiff neck or back.
- Be unusually tired.
- Have a different sounding cry from normal.
- Find it painful to look at a light.
- Be very irritable.

If your baby has meningitis she may develop a rash early on. The rash may become pink or purple and it will not go pale when you press the side of a glass against it. **If you ever see a rash like this on an adult or a child, seek immediate medical help. If you cannot contact a GP, take your baby to a hospital casualty department (A&E). However, if your baby is ill, don't wait for a rash to appear before getting help from your GP or hospital.**

One of the problems with meningitis is that early on, it can look as if your child has a fever. Although your GP will think about meningitis and probably test for it, a baby who is in the early stages may not show the signs of meningitis until some hours later. Don't be afraid to ask your GP about the meningitis signs to look out for. If your baby's condition seems to be getting worse call your GP back.

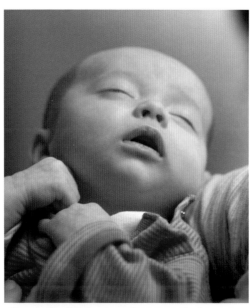

If your baby has colic, cuddle her so she feels secure

Colic

Colic is a term used to describe a particular type of crying.
- If your baby has colic she will look as if she is in a lot of pain.
- She may draw her knees up towards her stomach, clench her fists and screw up her face. This sort of crying usually starts when the baby is around three to four weeks old and is at its worse when the baby is about six to eight weeks old.
- Babies with colic cry for several hours at a time, often in the evenings.

- Sometimes you will be able to soothe your baby for a short while, but the crying soon starts again, for no obvious reason. In every other way, babies with colic are usually happy, healthy and developing normally.

Babies usually stop getting colic after they are three months old, though some babies can have it until they are about five months old.

How can I help my baby if she has colic?

Unfortunately there is not a lot you can do to help. However, you can try the following:
- If you are breastfeeding, check that she is finishing the first breast before starting on the second.
- Give your baby a warm bath.
- Cuddle her so she feels secure.
- Massage her feet.
- Let her suck a dummy.
- Give your baby colic drops or gripe water. You can buy these at a pharmacy.
- Lay her on your lap and gently rub her tummy in a clockwise direction.
- Try taking her for a walk or drive. If nothing helps, you need support, get someone to help you when your baby is crying and remember, colic will cause no lasting harm to your baby.
- Remember to look after yourself – for example, have a sleep in the afternoon so you are less tired in the evening.

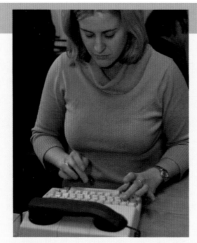

Further information

- National Childbirth Trust
- The Foundation for the Study of Infant Deaths
- Meningitis Research Foundation

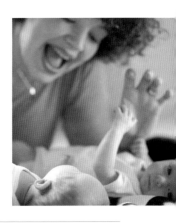

Chapter 16
Looking after yourself now you have a new baby

Sharon's story

Being at home during the first few weeks [after my son was born] were the most wonderful and yet exhausting days of my life – breastfeeding, after a difficult start went well and I was so much in love with my baby son that I did not mind the lack of sleep. I enjoyed breastfeeding so much that I ended up doing it for 15 months with both children – and I had only planned to do it for a couple of months.

I was very lucky in that the first few weeks after my daughter's birth were not too exhausting. I had also built up a network of local friends with children, through the National Childbirth Trust, and they helped out by looking after my son – bringing me cooked meals and lending me clothes. My son, being so young, still had daytime naps so we all used to have a sleep at the same time. My daughter was a very good sleeper so nights were easy to cope with.

My children are now five and three and we are really proud of their ability to communicate with different people – they seem to know instinctively how best to make themselves understood to friends, both deaf and hearing, and family. We feel that having positive Deaf parents has given them the gift of communication and as a result they are confident and sociable children.

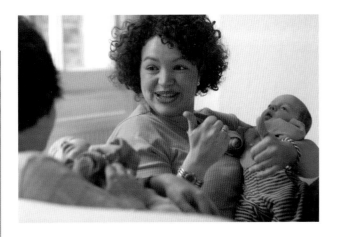

Getting support from your family and friends

Your family and friends can be a great source of support and help when you have a new baby and you should ask for as much support as you can. However, you may find that some hearing family members might be worried about how you will be able to manage to bring up a baby, particularly if your baby is hearing. They may worry about how your baby is going to learn to speak or how you will hear your baby crying.

You can reassure them that your hearing baby will hear spoken language when she spends time with members of the family and relatives, and when she is playing with other children. If your baby learns BSL from you she may well become bilingual.

If you have any concerns about your child's language development do discuss them with your GP, health visitor and other parents.

Important infomation

- Start exercising very gently in the first few weeks after you have had your baby.
- **Never** lie flat on your back and lift both legs in the air.
- **Never** lie flat on your back and do sit-ups with your feet held down.

This will put too much strain on your back and stomach muscles. Instead try pelvic floor exercises, pelvic tilting and rocking. Ask your midwife to show you how.

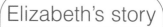

Elizabeth's story

After the birth of my baby in the hospital, a couple of nurses were very good to me and made a big effort. I found it hard at night because I was afraid I wouldn't hear my baby cry. I could sometimes hear that a baby was crying but couldn't distinguish if it was my baby or someone else's baby crying. I slept with the baby in bed with me instead.

When I got home, it was hard and I was trying to cope like all new mothers. The community midwife was fantastic – probably because by sheer coincidence she was hard of hearing too. So she knew just how to talk to me and we both understood each other perfectly.

My biggest fears while I was pregnant were, firstly, that I wouldn't be able to hear my child talk. Most children I come across talk very softly and I can't hear what they are saying and my fear was that it would be like that with my child. I'm not sure if it is genetic or learnt, but my child has a low, loud and clear voice – perfect for me. So that fear was unfounded. My child is also learning some basic sign language too.

Secondly, I was worried that something awful would happen in the night because I couldn't hear my baby cry. I bought a very good baby monitor with flashing lights. The lights alone are enough to wake me from a deep sleep – I think you become tuned into it – so whereas I might sleep through a thunderstorm, my child coughing through the night meant a few flashing lights on the monitor were enough to wake me up.*

So my two biggest fears were unfounded.

The positive side of being pregnant was having my child, which changed my life. I can't imagine being without my child in my life.

* Although flashing lights worked for Elizabeth, RNID recommends that you buy a monitor which also has a vibrating pad to wake you at night. See *Chapter 3 Finding out you are pregnant* for more information about baby monitors.

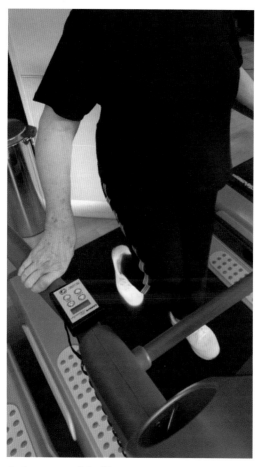

Ask your midwife to show you how to do postnatal exercises

What are postnatal exercises?

- These are exercises to help you get your body into shape after giving birth. You can start doing them a few weeks after you have had your baby. Ask your midwife if you can start doing them. The best way to learn them is to join a postnatal exercise class or ask your midwife to teach you. Your midwife will usually show you what to do and give you a list of exercises soon after the birth or before you are discharged from their care.
- Many NHS Trusts also have a physiotherapist who can give advice on postnatal exercises. If your baby is born in hospital, the physiotherapist will usually give you advice and a leaflet about postnatal exercises. You can ask to see them if you have questions or concerns.
- You will usually be given one set of exercises if you have had a vaginal birth and a different set of exercises if you have had a caesarean birth.

Lochia

- After birth you will lose some blood through your vagina. This can go on for several weeks. It comes from your womb – where the placenta was attached to the inside of the womb.
- You will bleed until the womb heals. At first the blood is bright red. You may have clots of blood. If they are as large as your fist, or you are worried about your blood loss, tell the midwife. The blood will gradually change to a brownish, more watery loss.
- It is best to use sanitary towels to avoid infection. Resting and looking after yourself will help you to recover more quickly.

How long should I wait before having sex after birth?

There are no rules about when to start having sex after you have given birth but if you are bleeding or having any discharge, you should ask your midwife or GP for advice about when to start. Don't feel pressurised into having sex if you are tired, or sore, or sex hurts or you don't feel like it. You should not have sex till you feel comfortable. You may find a lubricating cream helpful.

When should I start using contraception?

It is possible to get pregnant as early as three weeks after the birth of your baby because you may have started ovulating again. Ovulation is when you release an egg once a month from your ovaries. Get advice from your midwife or GP as soon as you can after your baby is born and before you start having sex again.

Can I get pregnant even if my periods have not started after giving birth?

Yes. Speak to your midwife or GP about using contraception.

Can I get pregnant if I am breastfeeding?

Yes. Even if you are breastfeeding, it may not stop you getting pregnant.

Useful tips

Don't expect too much of yourself in the first few weeks after birth. To begin with, you'll probably find that you want to concentrate on looking after your baby and yourself.

Before the birth, plan some ways you will be able to get support. Talk to friends and family so they understand the kind of support you want. Tell them you may change your mind after the birth.

You need to recover from the birth too. Try these tips:
- Give yourself as many breaks as possible and don't feel guilty about it.
- Sleep when your baby sleeps. If you can't sleep, at least lie down and rest.
- Eat regularly – 'ready-meals' save time and energy, but have some fresh fruit as well. Try a large sandwich and some soup, or pasta, whatever is quick and easy to do.
- Accept all offers of help – ironing, cooking, or shopping.
- Find out about local support groups such as parent and toddler groups.
- Don't overload yourself with too many visitors. If you do have visitors let them look after you.
- Don't try and do too much, too soon.

If you feel stressed, or worried about yourself or your baby, it is important to discuss your concerns with your partner or someone close to you. You can also speak to your midwife or health visitor.

What are the baby blues?

- Many new mothers get the baby blues around the third or fourth day after giving birth. It is common and quite normal.
- Baby blues make you feel weepy during the first week after your baby's birth.
- They last from a few days to just over a week and, although they may be upsetting, they are not normally serious and you usually soon stop feeling weepy.
- If you have the baby blues you may feel confused or disappointed because you are not feeling happy. You may find yourself worrying about things that don't normally bother you.

The important thing to remember is that the baby blues are very common and that

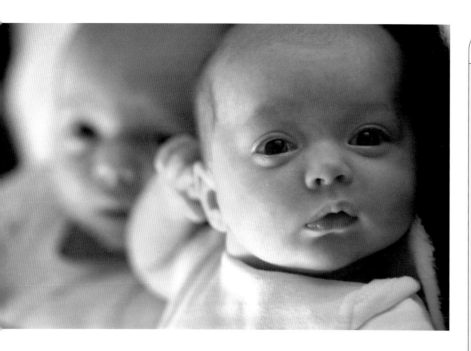

most women feel better very quickly. However, if you are feeling vulnerable, or you have had depression, or felt low in the past, you may find it more difficult to come to terms with being a mother and you may develop more serious postnatal depression.

What can be done to help?

- If you have the baby blues you need to get as much rest as possible. You should make sure that you have at least one proper rest, in bed, every day, in the first week or so after the baby is born.
- It is OK for you to feel upset and cry when you want to. You will need to explain this to your partner and family. This will help them support you. They need to understand that you have a real problem and should not keep telling you to cheer up.
- If you feel that you cannot cope at home with your baby after all the support you had in hospital try to get as much practical help as possible from your partner, family and friends. Ask them to do the housework and the

Katie's story

Deafness in parents need not be a barrier. The instincts we have as parents do all the work.

Farah's story

When I had my baby, I was exhausted and new to motherhood. Also, because it was traditional and common in my Asian culture for my husband's mum to stay with us and help me to settle into a routine with my baby, I found it particularly hard.

My mother-in-law meant well and cared for my baby, picking him up when he cried and allowing me to get extra sleep. However, there were times when I had my baby sleeping with me and I wanted to be there when he woke up, but because I couldn't hear my baby crying, or I was too exhausted, my mother-in-law just came into the room to pick him up and left the room. I felt at that point, the bonding between my baby and me was fading away and that my mother-in-law was taking over without asking me first. I wasn't sure whether it was because I'm Deaf or because my mother-in-law felt I should have as much rest as possible. I only wanted to get into the routine of being a mother and was looking forward to spending lots of time with my baby. However, I felt frustrated and the only time I had with my baby was when I was breastfeeding, which I valued each time.

I remember, once I had a health check-up with the GP and health visitor. I decided to take my baby with me for the first time in my car. It felt so odd. I had a baby seat and found it hard to check on my baby whilst driving, as my rear view mirror wasn't large enough to see my baby at

shopping so you can then concentrate on yourself and your baby.
- Usually, you won't need to take any medicine although if you have trouble sleeping your doctor may suggest a short course of sleeping pills. But take care if you are breastfeeding as you may be too sleepy in the night to cope with breastfeeding and will need help.
- Baby blues usually disappear after a few days. However, if they get worse you should see your doctor in case you have developed postnatal depression.

the back. So I e-mailed the Deaf parenting e-mail group*, asking for suggestions from other deaf parents as to how to resolve this. On their suggestion I bought an additional large rear view mirror which I positioned so I could see my baby at the back of the car. It worked very well.**

Anyway back to the appointment. I then did a bit of shopping with my baby and had a nice walk, a complete break from staying at home and found it refreshing and calming. When I got home, my mother-in-law was worried and almost panicking, not knowing where I was and whether I was able to cope with the baby alone without support. I told her that I had managed fine. I had to be careful in dealing with her. I think for some reason, hearing people don't realise how capable deaf parents can be in caring for their baby and we need to show them that we are just as capable as anyone else.

It is important to communicate your feelings with your partner. It is OK to feel frustrated but you are not alone and it can happen to many new mums, deaf or hearing.

*See *Chapter 21 Further information* for details.
**Have a look at RNID's factsheet *Cars and public transport – information for deaf and hard of hearing people.* You can buy mirrors from motoring shops and baby shops.

What is the difference between the baby blues and postnatal depression?

Postnatal depression is a serious mental health condition that some mothers can get after they have had a baby. Mild postnatal depression is quite common. More serious postnatal depression is quite rare. Postnatal depression is quite different and separate from the baby blues. It is also more serious.

Why do some mothers get the baby blues or postnatal depression?

It is not always easy to explain why some mothers get postnatal depression.
- Researchers think it is linked to the all the emotions you go through when you are pregnant, give birth and are faced with the responsibility of being a mother.
- The physical changes, and possibly the hormonal changes, that your body goes through, probably play a part.
- Many mothers find having a new baby a complete shock. They may worry both before and after the baby is born about how they will cope.
- Also, although it is important for you to rest after you have had a baby, in reality you may find this very difficult.

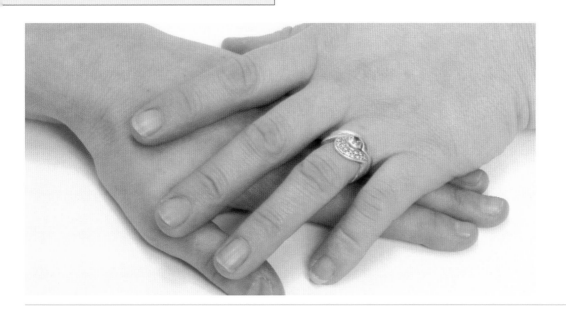

What are the signs of postnatal depression?

If you have postnatal depression you may:
- Feel unable to cope.
- Feel guilty or inadequate.
- Have sleeping and eating difficulties.
- Have little interest in sex.
- Feel irritable.
- Get panic attacks.
- Find it hard to concentrate.
- Feel rejected by your partner, family, friends or even your baby.

What help is available?

- Postnatal depression is a real illness. Remember that it is not your fault and that you can get help.
- Speak to your midwife or health visitor. They will advise you to see your doctor who may suggest counselling and/or anti-depressant drugs.
- Many mothers find that support groups can be very helpful.
- You will also need to get as much rest as possible and ask for support from your partner, family and friends. Talking to a member of your family, or a friend, who can listen to you and accept how you feel can be very helpful.
- Women do recover with treatment.

You may not have postnatal depression but may feel upset and worried about the whole experience of childbirth and becoming a mother. Speak to your midwife, heath visitor or GP about your worries.

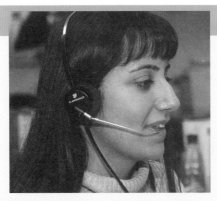

Further information

- Association for Post-Natal Illness
- Homestart
- Maternity Alliance
- National Childbirth Trust
- One Parent Families
- www.parentcentre.gov.uk
- WellBeing

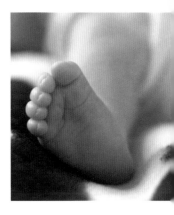

Chapter 17
Becoming a father

Finding out you're going to be a father

When you first find out you're going to be a father you will probably feel a range of emotions. You might feel excited, horrified, full of joy, frightened, on top of the world, angry, sad, or overwhelmed. Everyone feels differently – there's no right way to feel.

You will probably have lots of questions yourself. Ask your partner if she wants you to go along with her to any appointments she has with the GP or midwife, so you can ask questions. You can also contact any of the organisations in *Chapter 21 Further information*. They can all help fathers and fathers-to-be, as well as mothers.

You can also look at the other chapters in this book with your partner. Use this book to help you discuss ideas.

Can I be present when my baby is born?

Yes, so long as your partner wants you to be there, you can be present throughout labour and birth. Lots of fathers find it an amazing experience, however not everyone feels the same way about it. Some men can find it frightening, they don't like seeing their partner in pain and it can make them feel helpless. Some men find they feel like a spare part and don't know how best to help. Find out what your partner would like you to do before she goes into labour.

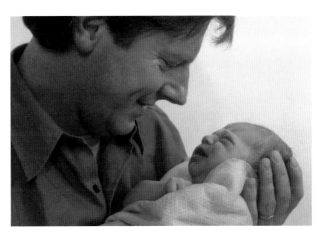

Try asking other fathers about how they felt when their partners were giving birth. It can also help if you prepare yourself and make sure you have some idea of what to expect when your partner is in labour. Men can go along with their partners to antenatal classes so this is a good way to find out more.
Discuss your partner's birth plan with her and ask her to write down what she wants you to do during labour and birth.

Sam's story

Communication is especially important because when my wife was going through pregnancy and experiencing physical body changes, including hormone changes and mood swings, I found it difficult, especially as a man, to understand what she was going through. At times, she was emotional, at times she needed a hug or something to be done, sometimes I didn't know where I stood with her especially with her mood swings. I am sure many women would understand how she felt but me, as a man, I felt hopeless. However, to support my wife and to share anxiety, concerns and excitement that pregnancy brought us, I decided to do lots of reading on pregnancy, that my wife lent me, but I found most books too waffly.

How can I help my partner when she's in labour?

There are lots of different ways you can help your partner:

- You can help her with her breathing and relaxation techniques. You can learn what to do at antenatal classes.
- You can give her physical or emotional support when she asks for it. For example, she might want you to massage her, or support her when she tries out new positions. You could help her operate the gas and air machine or just encourage her.
- She may just want you to be with her and hold her hand.
- You can help make sure her wishes are followed.
- You can help 'relay' information to her.

Kevin's story

We contacted the Deaf Parenting Project at DPPi* and they've been very helpful. They have a library with various booklets and information sheets for Deaf parents. They also searched on the Internet for some extra information to help us with our home birth preparation.

For our home birth, I wrote a letter to the local NHS Trust's Midwifery Unit specifically requesting that they support our choice and provide a midwife who could work with BSL interpreters or write lots of notes for us. They did provide this.

After moving house at week 36, we saw our new community midwife for an antenatal check. The next day, she dropped off a home birth kit at our home. No fuss. We were prepared to stand up for our rights and instead we found full support.

It was a bit frustrating that the NHS's contracted interpreting agency could not supply a BSL interpreter easily – they needed at least four weeks' notice. As it turned out the labour and our daughter's birth was a brilliant experience – with just ourselves and the two midwives. An intimate event without the distraction of using a BSL interpreter. Both midwives communicated with us by writing and then I would translate to/from my wife in sign language.

*Disability, Pregnancy and Parenthood international. You will find their contact details in *Chapter 21 Further information*.

How can I help with a newborn baby?

There are lots of things you can do to help your partner look after your new baby:

- Take time off work in the first few weeks if you can. For information about paternity leave, see *Chapter 18 Working parents – maternity and paternity rights*.
- Use this time to give as much practical help as you can – change nappies, do the shopping, cooking and housework.
- Support your partner if she is breastfeeding, or help with preparing bottles and feeding, if she is bottle feeding.
- Help your partner bath your baby.
- Answer telephone/textphone calls and look after visitors.

Remember, becoming a parent will be a new, exhausting and exciting time for both of you. Take time to care for each other and share your feelings and worries.

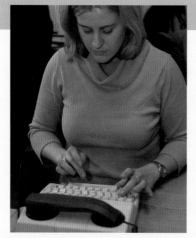

Further information

- Maternity Alliance
- National Childbirth Trust
- www.parentcentre.gov.uk

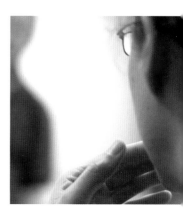

Chapter 18

Working parents – maternity and paternity rights

Below we have answered some of the more commonly asked questions about rights for pregnant women and new parents who are working. This is only a brief look and you should contact one of the organisations listed in *Further information* at the end of this chapter for more advice.

Can I take time-off during pregnancy for antenatal care?

Yes. If you are working you have the right to take paid time-off work for antenatal care (see *Chapter 7 Antenatal care* for more information).

Do I get extra health and safety protection at work?

Yes.
- If you are pregnant, have recently given birth or are breastfeeding, you have the right to extra health and safety protection at work. This means your employer must make sure that being at work does not put your health, or your baby's health, at risk.
- Your employer must remove or adapt anything that can risk your health or your unborn child's health.
- If they can't do this they must adapt your working conditions, or the hours you work, so you are no longer at risk.
- If this is not possible your employer must offer you a suitable alternative job.
- If they can't offer you a suitable alternative job, they should suspend you on full pay until your health, or your baby's health, would no longer be at risk at work.

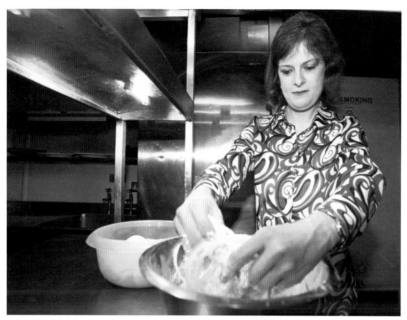

You have the right to extra health and safety protection at work

What is maternity leave?

If you are working and pregnant you will be able to take maternity leave. This is paid time-off from work with the right to return to work at the end of your leave. Your employer has to give you this leave by law.

There are two sorts of maternity leave depending on how long you have been working for your employer – **ordinary maternity leave** and **additional maternity leave**. You may be entitled to ordinary maternity leave or you may be entitled to ordinary maternity leave plus additional maternity leave.

What is ordinary maternity leave?
- Ordinary maternity leave is 26 weeks leave from work.
- You have the right to return to your job at the end of the 26 weeks.
- It doesn't matter how many hours you work or how long you have worked for your employer.
- You can start your leave up to 11 weeks before your baby is due or you can work right up to the date your baby is due to be born unless:
    - You are ill, or away from work, due to your pregnancy, in the last four weeks of your pregnancy. In this case your employer can choose to start your maternity leave even if

you are only off sick for one day.
- Your baby is born before the day you were planning to start your leave. In this case your leave will start on the day after the birth.
- You may be entitled to Statutory Maternity Pay or Maternity Allowance during ordinary maternity leave.

How do I tell my employer that I want to take maternity leave (give notice)?
To get maternity leave you must give your employer the following information, in, or before, the 15th week before your baby is due (if you are asked to, you must put it in writing).
- That you are pregnant.
- The week you expect to give birth.
- The date you plan to start ordinary maternity leave.

You can change the date you start your maternity leave but you must give your employer at least 28 days notice.

What is additional maternity leave?
- If you have worked for your employer for 26 weeks by the 15th week before your baby is due to be born you can also take additional maternity leave.
- Additional maternity leave lasts for 26 weeks and starts the day after your ordinary maternity leave ends.
- You have the right to return to your job at the end of the 52 weeks.
- 26 weeks ordinary maternity leave + 26 weeks additional maternity leave = 52 weeks (one year).
- Additional maternity leave is usually a period of unpaid leave.

When you go back to work after additional maternity leave you have the right to return to the same job you were doing before. But if your employer can show that this is not practical you have the right to a suitable alternative job, on similar terms and conditions.

What if I work in a small firm?
If you work for a firm that employs five people, or fewer, you still have the right to additional maternity leave, but your employer may not need to keep your job

open or offer you a very similar job. You should get advice from one of the organisations listed at the end of this chapter.

How can I take extra leave?

You cannot take extra maternity leave, but you can take what is known as **parental leave** when your maternity leave comes to an end. We give more information later in this chapter.

What is maternity pay?

Maternity pay is money you may be able to get from the government whilst you are on maternity leave. There are two sorts of maternity pay – **Statutory Maternity Pay** and **Maternity Allowance**.

Statutory Maternity Pay
Statutory Maternity Pay lasts 26 weeks. Your employer pays it to you. Your employer will be able to tell you if you are entitled to it, or contact one of the organisations listed at the end of this chapter.

How much is Statutory Maternity Pay?
For the first six weeks you get 90% of your average pay. After that you get £102.80 per week for 20 weeks, or 90% of your average earnings if you earn less than £102.80 a week.

Maternity Allowance
- You may be able to get Maternity Allowance if you don't qualify for Statutory Maternity Pay. Jobcentre Plus pays Maternity Allowance for 26 weeks.
- Ask your local Jobcentre Plus for information or contact one of the organisations listed at the end of this chapter.

How much is Maternity Allowance?
Maternity Allowance is £102.80 for 26 weeks or 90% of your average earnings if you earn less than £102.80 a week.

Incapacity Benefit

If you do not qualify for Maternity Allowance you may be able to claim Incapacity Benefit. Contact your local Jobcentre Plus for information.

Maternity policies

Your employer may have a **maternity policy**. This policy may only give you the basic statutory maternity rights but it may also give you some extra rights.

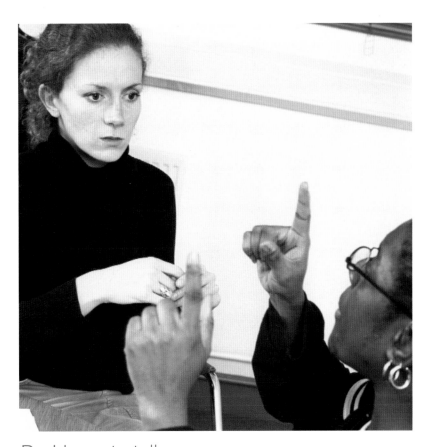

Do I have to tell my employers I am coming back to work?

Ordinary maternity leave
When you are on ordinary maternity leave you do not need to contact your employer to tell them you are going back to work at the end of it. It is your right to return to work to exactly the same job that you were doing before you went on leave. Your employer should write to you with the date when your ordinary maternity leave ends.

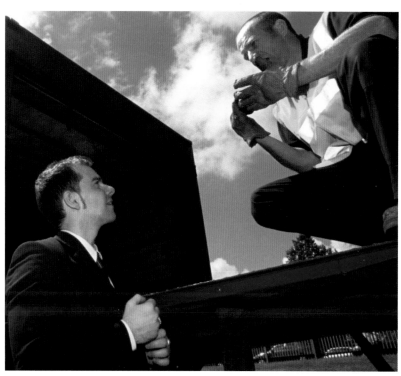

Find out about paternity leave

What is parental leave?

- Parental leave is designed to give both mothers and fathers more time with their young children.
- By law each parent is allowed to take 13 weeks unpaid leave for each child they have up until their child's fifth birthday. If your child is entitled to Disability Living Allowance (DLA) you can take up to 18 weeks parental leave until your child's 18th birthday. This leave is also available to parents who adopt a baby.
- Have a look at your own employer's parental leave scheme as it could be more flexible or more generous than the parental leave you are allowed by law.
- Usually you need to have worked for a year for your employer before you are entitled to take parental leave. You can take parental leave at the end of your maternity leave as long as you give your employer 21 days' notice.
- Your employer can ask that you do not take the leave immediately, for up to six months, if they think it will disrupt their business.
- Parental leave is usually *unpaid*.
- Parental leave is not the same as paternity leave. If you are a new father you can take some of your parental leave at the time of the birth of your baby if for some reason you are unable to take paternity leave.

Additional maternity leave

If you take the 26 weeks of additional maternity leave, you do not need to tell your employer you are going back to work. They must assume you are going to take it and write to you with the date when it ends.

What if I do not want to take all the leave I am entitled to?

You can end your maternity leave early by giving your employer 28 days' notice.

Can I return to work but do fewer hours or different hours?

If you ask to change your hours because of childcare your employer must consider your request seriously. They can only refuse you if they have good business reasons. You should put your request in writing and your employer must follow correct procedures when considering your request.

What is paternity leave and who can get it?

- Paternity leave is for fathers of new babies, or partners of women with new babies, who have been born after 6 April 2003. If someone adopts a child, their partner can also take paternity leave.
- The father should either be the biological father of your baby, or your husband or partner. They should also be planning to be involved in bringing up your baby.
- They must have worked continuously for their employer for 26 weeks up to the 15th week before the baby is due.

How much paternity leave can fathers take?

Fathers can take from one to two weeks. If they take two weeks, these have to be taken together.

Is paternity leave paid?

Fathers, partners and adopters are entitled to Statutory Paternity Pay (SPP) from their employers if they qualify. Fathers will have to give their employer notice that they are planning to take paternity leave, by the end of the 15th week before the baby is due to be born, and if this is not possible, then as soon as it is reasonably practical.

How much is Statutory Paternity Pay?

SPP is paid at a rate of £102.80 a week or 90% of the father's average earnings if he earns less than £102.80 a week.

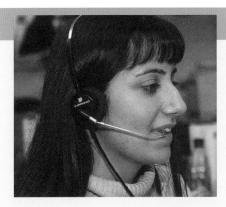

Further information

- www.dti.gov.uk
- Jobcentre Plus
- Maternity Alliance
- Working families
- www.tiger.gov.uk

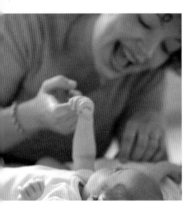

Chapter 19
Your rights under the Disability Discrimination Act (1995)

There are now laws in the UK, which aim to ensure that you are not discriminated against as deaf parents, or parents-to-be. In this section we look at one of these laws – the Disability Discrimination Act 1995 (DDA).

We have also included some information about the Human Rights Act (1998).

If you want to find out more about these laws contact RNID or any of the organisations listed at the end of this chapter for more information.

What is the DDA?

The DDA is a law. It was introduced in 1995 to stop discrimination against disabled people as customers. It seeks to give disabled people equal rights and access to goods, facilities and services. The DDA says that service providers are not allowed to treat disabled or deaf people less favourably because of their disability.

What is discrimination?

The DDA says that discrimination is when service providers treat disabled people less favourably because of their disability and they cannot justify this.

Jennifer's story

My health visitor is great as she has the right attitude, she is very patient with me and has booked interpreters whenever I ask her. I think it helps if you know your rights, such as getting an interpreter, or birth options.

Are deaf people covered by the DDA?

Yes.
- Anyone who meets the Act's definition of disability is covered by the DDA. The Act defines disability as "a physical or mental impairment which has a substantial and long term adverse effect on [the person's] ability to carry out normal day to day activities".
- An "inability to hold a conversation with someone talking in a normal voice" or an "inability to hear and understand another person speaking clearly over the voice telephone" counts as a substantial 'adverse effect' under the Act. This means that deaf people are covered by the DDA.
- The Act also allows the effect of background noise on your deafness to be taken into account.
- Even if you use a hearing aid, your hearing *without* the hearing aid is what counts.

Are GP surgeries and hospitals covered by the DDA?

Yes. Under the DDA, 'service providers' includes most companies or organisations that offer goods, facilities or services to the general public. It does not matter whether the services are free or paid for. This means that the DDA covers:

- GP surgeries.
- Family planning clinics.
- NHS hospitals.
- Private hospitals.
- Antenatal classes.

How can the DDA help deaf people?

The DDA makes it unlawful for a service provider, for example, a hospital, to treat you less favourably than they would treat a hearing person, or a person with a different disability. The DDA says there are four types of unlawful discrimination:

- Refusing to give you a service because you are deaf. For example, a GP surgery refusing to accept you as a new patient because you are deaf.
- Not making a reasonable adjustment, for example refusing to take a call made via RNID Typetalk.
- Offering a lower standard of service or providing a service in a worse manner, such as making you wait longer for an appointment than a hearing person.
- Providing a service on worse terms, such as asking you for a deposit for a private antenatal class, although hearing people do not have to pay a deposit, because the organiser believes that because you are deaf you are less likely to go to the classes.

Do service providers have to change the way they work?

Service providers may have to change the way they provide services to make sure that disabled people can make use of them. Service providers, such as hospitals or GP surgeries, will have to do this if it is 'impossible or unreasonably difficult' for you to access their services because you are deaf. This is known as the 'duty to make reasonable adjustments'.

What sort of 'reasonable adjustments' would a service provider have to make?

Service providers, for example, a health clinic, may be required to provide extra aids or services so that you can access a service more easily, for example:

- Deaf awareness training for staff.
- Written information, such as a leaflet or guide.
- A speech-to-text service.
- Induction loop or infrared systems.
- Subtitled and signed videos.
- Information displayed on a computer screen.
- Textphones, telephone amplifiers and inductive couplers.
- Teletext displays.
- Videophones.
- Fire alarm systems for deaf people.
- Qualified BSL/English interpreters or lipspeakers.

Does the service provider have to provide everything I need?

The service provider has to do what is 'reasonable'. This will depend on a number of things, including the type of service provider, how big or small they are, how much money and other resources they have, and the effect that your being deaf has on you.

For example:
- How practical is it for your GP surgery, to meet your needs? For example, how easy would it be for them to book a BSL/English interpreter at short notice?
- Will the adjustment help you access healthcare services? For example, will you be able to understand your midwife's advice if you use a lipspeaker?
- How much would it cost to install a permanent induction loop?
- What has the service provider already spent on making adjustments?

This is not a complete list but it should give you an idea of some of the reasons why a service provider may not have to provide everything you need.

My GP surgery has a textphone but no one seems to know how to use it

Under the DDA, service providers must make sure that the adjustments they make are effective. For example:
- If your GP has a textphone, staff in the surgery should know how to use it.
- If a hospital provides a BSL/English interpreter, they should be suitably qualified.

Do I have to pay for the 'adjustment'?

It is up to service providers to organise and pay for 'adjustments'. If the additional service, for example a BSL/English interpreter, is a 'reasonable adjustment', then you do not have to pay for it. You should not have to pay for any service that is usually available free to hearing people.

Justifying discrimination

Like all laws the DDA can be quite complicated. For example, occasionally a service provider, such as a hospital, is allowed to treat a disabled person less favourably. This is called 'justification'. The DDA says that a service provider can only do this if certain conditions are met.

If you want to find out more about the DDA, see RNID's factsheet *The Disability Discrimination Act 1995 (DDA) – a guide for deaf and hard of hearing customers*.

What to do if you think you have been discriminated against

If you have been discriminated against, you may be able to take legal action under the DDA. Get advice from one of the organisations listed at the end of this chapter.

What is the Human Rights Act (1998)?

The Human Rights Act (1998) gives everyone, including disabled and deaf people, extra rights in law. If you are not happy with the treatment you have received from an NHS Trust you may also be able to bring a claim under the Human Rights Act. For more information see RNID's factsheet *The Human Rights Act (1998) – information for deaf and hard of hearing people*. You can also contact the organisations listed at the end of this chapter to get advice.

Sam's story

Looking back* it was really a bad time for us. The hospital didn't have any deaf awareness and none of the staff were aware of our needs. I really wish I had complained about the service we received compared with other parents. We came home and were so happy and busy, concentrating on our new baby that we didn't complain. I wish we complained at the time.

* You can read about Sam and Rosie's experience of labour, birth and on the maternity ward in *Chapter 10 Labour and birth* and *Chapter 11 Your baby's first few days*.

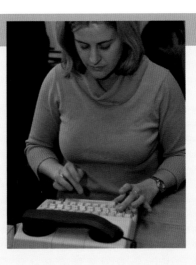

Further information

- The Association for Improvements in the Maternity Services
- British Deaf Association
- Citizens Advice Bureau (CAB)
- Community Legal Service
- Disability Law Service
- Disability Rights Commission
- Law centres
- Patient Advocacy Liaison Service
- RNID Casework Service
- RNID Information Line

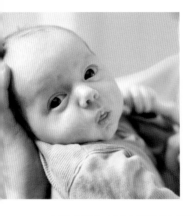

Chapter 20
Information for health professionals

Throughout this book you will find stories from deaf mothers and mothers-to-be. We have also included some stories from deaf fathers. Although many have had positive care from health professionals, many others found the lack of deaf awareness distressing at a time when they particularly needed support. We hope that these stories and tips for better communication will encourage you to look at your own policies and practices for working with deaf parents and parents-to-be.

How do deaf people communicate?

Deaf people choose to communicate in different ways depending on their level of deafness, for example, someone who is severely deaf may need a BSL/English interpreter to follow what is being said but may be able to speak clearly.

> "When I was pregnant, the professionals would always try to talk to my hearing partner instead of to me, but my husband would tell them to talk directly to me as it was me who was having the baby, not him."

- Some people with a **mild** hearing loss might use a hearing aid or find lipreading helpful.
- People with **moderate** hearing loss will have difficulty hearing what is said without a hearing aid, particularly somewhere noisy.
- People who are **severely** deaf may have difficulty following what is being said even with a hearing aid. Many lipread and some use sign language or speech-to-text.
- Some, but not all, people who are **profoundly** deaf may find that hearing aids are of little benefit to them. They may use sign language, speech-to-text or lipread.

Communication services

There is a wide range of communication services available to help deaf and hearing people communicate with each other. Remember, always ask the deaf person you are working with what type of support they would prefer. You will often need to book several weeks in advance to ensure you get a service. We give lots of useful information below to help you book a communication service.

- A **BSL/English interpreter** interprets from one language to the other. In the UK this will usually be from BSL to spoken or written English, or spoken or written English to BSL. If you have a videophone, for example, in your surgery, it may be appropriate to use a video interpreting service.

- **Lipspeakers** repeat what a hearing person or speaker is saying, without using their voice, so that deaf and hard of hearing people can lipread them.
- **Speech-to-text reporters** (also known as **palantypists** or **stenographers**) type every word that is spoken using a special keyboard. Everything that is said appears on a computer screen.
- **Electronic notetakers** (or **SpeedText® operators**) type a *summary* of what has been said. This appears on a computer screen for the deaf person to read.
- **Notetakers** are trained to take accurate and clear notes for deaf and hard of hearing people.
- **Interpreters** or **communicator guides for deafblind people** help hearing and deafblind people communicate with each other.

Below we have given you some general tips to help you when working with deaf mothers. Lots of them have been provided by health professionals with experience of working with deaf mothers.

Tips for better communication with deaf mothers

- Don't shout.
- Don't speak with your back to the mother.
- Always introduce yourself and others to the mother.
- Think about where you stand. Make sure the mother does not have to strain to see you or other staff.
- Make a note of whether the mother is deaf or hard of hearing, and her preferred method of communication, in her case notes, care plans and midwives' notes and make sure all staff are aware of this.
- If a mother uses BSL keep an A-Z fingerspelling chart, sign language chart or pen and paper handy. You can get fingerspelling charts from RNID. Make time so the mother can teach you some fingerspelling.
- If the mother's first or preferred

language is BSL, remember English may be her second or even third language. She may find understanding English very difficult. Write and speak in plain English. If you have to use medical terms explain what they mean.

- Always ensure patient confidentiality. Only ask a family member or friend to interpret if the mother gives her permission first – record this in her notes.
- Make sure you know how to get hold of a BSL/English interpreter, lipspeaker, or other form of communication support, including those available during out-of-hours or in an emergency, or make prior arrangements. Write these details down.
- You should tell the mother about your services, her treatment, medicine and possible side-effects in a way that meets her needs. This might mean using a BSL/English interpreter, if available, or providing information written in plain English and/or clear diagrams.
- Whenever possible, back up what you have told the mother with visual and written information so that she can read it later.
- Make sure that the mother understands any information you have given her and that she is not just agreeing to appear polite.
- Identify all staff who have had deaf awareness training. If possible assign a deaf aware midwife to the mother.
- Try and talk to the mother in a quiet room where there will be less background noise.
- Tap the mother on her arm, between the wrist and elbow, or wave your hand in front of her to let her know that you are there, but don't overdo it.
- If you are collecting a mother from a waiting area take her to the room where the appointment is, rather than just walking away.
- Make sure you have fitted special equipment for deaf people, or have equipment available for them to use, for example, induction loop or infrared systems and textphones.

"I don't feel that I had enough information given to me when I was pregnant, and this made me nervous."

Contact RNID Sound Advantage for more information about equipment.

"I have two hearing sons. I remember with my second child that when I saw the health visitor I couldn't understand her and so she tried to talk to my older son instead of directly to me. I sent the boys off to play so that she would talk to me instead. Sometimes professionals who have no deaf awareness use hearing children as interpreters and it's not right."

- Talk to the mother about equipment she can use in the home, such as baby monitors for deaf people, before she leaves hospital.
- If you are running antenatal or postnatal classes always explain first, then demonstrate.
- If videos are available try to get ones which are signed and/or subtitled.
- Explain the layout of the room before delivery. It takes time but can make it seem less frightening.
- During labour try and make sure that only one person is speaking at any one time.
- Mothers do not always have their eyes open during labour. This will make it impossible for them to see an interpreter or lipread you. You may have to use tactile signs, for example, 'press' if the mother needs to push,

'tap', if she has to stop pushing. Work out the best ones to use with the mother and make sure you use the same signs throughout pregnancy and labour.

- If the mother is tired or anxious, or has been given pain relief or drugs such as pethidine or entonox, this may affect her concentration.
- Ask the mother about the signs she would prefer to use during labour. Use these consistently during the antenatal period.
- If you have to insert an IV drip, remember that deaf mothers use their hands to sign.
- If the mother's partner is deaf make sure you meet their communication needs as well.
- Be aware of your legal responsibilities as a service provider under the Disability Discrimination Act (1995) and the Human Rights Act (1998). You must not treat deaf or other disabled people less favourably because of their hearing loss or other disability, and you may also have to make a reasonable adjustment to help a deaf person use your service. For more information, have a look at *Chapter 19 Your rights under the Disability Discrimination Act (1995)*.

Working with a mother who uses a hearing aid(s)

You can find out more about the different sort of hearing aids available and how they work by looking at RNID's leaflet *All about hearing aids*.

- You should make a note in the mother's care plan that she is a hearing aid user and let all staff know.
- Ensure that the maternity wards and delivery areas keep a supply of batteries suitable for the different sorts of hearing aids available.
- Mothers lying on their side may be covering their aid, which will make it harder for them to hear you.
- If a mother has an epidural she can keep her hearing aid(s) in.
- If the mother has a caesarean section reassure her that she does not have to remove her hearing aid(s) until she has been anaesthetised. Most caesarean section operations can be done with epidurals rather than a general anaesthetic so the mother can stay awake.
- Hearing aids should be kept in the recovery room.

Lipreading

Below you will find specific information to help you communicate with mothers who lipread. We also tell you more about booking a lipspeaker. RNID can also give you more information about lipreading and lipspeakers. Have a look at our leaflet *Lipreading and lipspeaking*.

Making it easier for someone to lipread you

- Find a suitable environment with good lighting, away from noise and distractions.
- Sit or stand at the same level as the mother, and three to six feet away (one to two metres).
- Face the light, or your face will be in shadow.
- Make sure the mother is looking at you before you speak.
- Introduce the topic of conversation.

- Speak clearly at a moderate pace without raising your voice or over-emphasising your speech.
- Use natural facial expressions, gestures and body language.
- Keep your face visible. Do not put your hands near it or wear sunglasses – and do not turn away while you are talking.
- Use plain English and repeat or rephrase something if the mother finds it difficult to follow.
- Check that the mother can follow you. Be patient as it takes time to communicate.
- Don't shine a light into the mother's eyes as this will make it difficult for her to look at your face.

Rosie's story

You will find Rosie's story about the birth of her first child in earlier chapters in this book. Since then, she has had twins.

When I was pregnant second time round I contacted the midwife and raised my concerns of my poor past experiences. She suggested that I contact the Director of Midwifery, which I did, and we arranged two deaf awareness training sessions with over 30 midwives.

During the training I got an excellent reception. Many of the midwives had a lot of fun learning the signs. I also made sure that I told them of my past experiences and how they could improve in communication with me as well as any future deaf mums.

When I went into labour, all the midwives on duty were very polite and attentive. I had very effective communication right from the start to the end. The anaesthetist who did my epidural was so nice and spoke very slowly. All these positive experiences made me enjoy my labour even more.

On the postnatal ward I was treated as if I was in a hotel. I had my own room and many of the midwives gave me excellent and encouraging support. I was very happy during my three night stay and I was rather disappointed when I left the hospital to go home!

Working with a lipspeaker

Lipspeakers repeat what a hearing person is saying, without using their voice, so that deaf and hard of hearing people can lipread them.

- Try and give the lipspeaker background information, in advance if possible, so that they can prepare themselves about the subject matter and any specialist words or phrases that may be used. If you can't do this because of client confidentiality, try and speak to them before they go in to the assignment.

> "I've given birth to three children, and with each child the first question by every professional usually has been, "Can the baby hear?". As if that's the most important thing. What matters is not deafness, but whether the baby is healthy and happy."

- It is important to book a suitably qualified lipspeaker. There are two levels of lipspeaking – Level 2 and Level 3. Only Level 3 lipspeakers are qualified to work in medical settings. You can ask for advice when making booking.
- All qualified registered lipspeakers are bound by a code of practice which means they must keep all information on assignments strictly confidential.

Remember

- If you wear a face mask the mother won't be able to lipread you.
- If she is anxious or tired this may interfere with her lipreading.
- Some birth positions are difficult to lipread from. Midwives may have to work in pairs.

Booking a lipspeaker
You will need to book as far in advance as possible – preferably two to three weeks.

To book a lipspeaker contact:

- **RNID Information Line.**
- **Council for the Advancement of Communication with Deaf People.**
- **The Association of Lipspeakers.**

You will find contact details in *Chapter 21 Further information* at the end of this book.

British Sign Language (BSL)

Many people who are born deaf or become deaf early in life use sign language to communicate. It is difficult to say how many people in the UK use BSL as their first or preferred language – current estimates suggest 50,000-70,000. In March 2003 the government recognised BSL as a language in its own right.

BSL developed naturally as languages do. It uses both manual and non-manual components – handshapes and movements, facial expression, and shoulder movement. BSL is structured in a completely different way from English, and like any language, it has its own grammar.

People who use BSL also use fingerspelling. Certain words – usually names of people and places – are spelled out on fingers. Fingerspelling alone is not sign language but it can be very useful when communicating with deaf signers.

If you would like to learn BSL contact the RNID Information Line for more information about classes in your area.

Tips for working with a BSL/English interpreter

- Make sure you book a BSL/English interpreter who is suitably qualified. Ask for advice when making your booking.

- Speak directly to the mother, not the interpreter.
- Do not say anything that you don't want interpreted. The interpreter will interpret everything that you say.
- Speak as you normally would and use normal facial expressions.
- Let the mother and interpreter decide where they would like to sit so that it is easy for the mother to see the interpreter.
- Remember the interpreter may have to get on the floor to enable the mother to see them.
- Use a room with good lighting so that the mother can see you and the interpreter clearly.
- If there are more than three people in the room make it clear at the start of the meeting/discussion that only one person speaks at any one time.
- Remember that the interpreter is a few words behind the speaker. Allow the interpreter time to finish before asking questions or starting a discussion.
- At times the interpreter may need to interrupt whoever is speaking to ask for clarification.
- Interpreters need a break after about half an hour.
- It is a good idea to send the interpreter background information at least two weeks before the assignment so that they know what to expect and can prepare, for example, topics and terminology to be discussed. If this is not possible due to patient confidentiality then discuss what the meeting is about before the interpreter enters the room.
- Interpreters have a strict code of practice and everything that is said in an assignment is strictly confidential. They cannot give advice or opinions whilst working with you.

Booking a BSL/English interpreter
- You can book a face-to-face BSL/English interpreter or a video interpreter. You may find that it is easier to get a video interpreter at short notice but there will be situations where it is more suitable to use an interpreter who can actually be in the room with you and the mother. You will need access to a videophone and

ISDN2 line in order to use a video interpreter. Contact RNID for more information about buying and using a videophone and for information about working with a BSL/English interpreter.

- It may be appropriate to book a female interpreter.
- If possible try to book the same interpreter throughout the pregnancy and labour.
- Make sure you book a BSL/English interpreter who is suitably qualified. You can get advice when making your booking.
- Book an interpreter as far in advance as possible, at least three weeks.
- Because labour is unpredictable, it can be hard to book an interpreter who can be there just when you need them. If you need an interpreter at short notice because of an emergency this may be difficult to arrange. There is no easy way round this but it will help if you plan ahead as far in advance as possible and phone your local interpreting service long before a woman's labour is due to start. Ask them for advice as different areas may have different emergency interpreting systems and solutions.

How to book a BSL/English interpreter

- Use an agency or
- Book directly with a freelance interpreter – someone who works for themselves.

Finding an agency

You can contact any of the following:

- RNID Communication Services (via RNID Information Line)
- Council for the Advancement of Communication with Deaf People
- Scottish Association of Sign Language Interpreters
- Wales Council for the Deaf

It is a good idea to open an account with an interpreting agency.

You will find all contact details in *Chapter 21 Further information* at the end of this book.

Booking a freelance interpreter

- Contact the Council for the Advancement of Communication with Deaf People for details of freelance interpreters.
- Ask the mother if she knows of any freelance interpreters she feels comfortable working with.

Booking a video interpreter

Contact:

- RNID Video Interpreting (contact RNID Information Line)
- Council for the Advancement of Communication with Deaf People

Further information

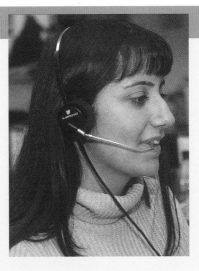

- The Association of Lipspeakers
- British Deaf Association
- Council for the Advancement of Communication with Deaf People
- Hearing Concern
- RNID Information Line (including information on RNID Video Interpreting)
- Scottish Association of Sign Language Interpreters
- Wales Council for the Deaf

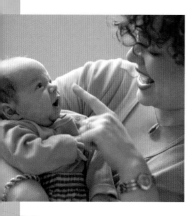

Chapter 21
Further information

At the end of each chapter in this book we have listed organisations where you can get further information. You will find all the contact details below.

Some of the organisations hire and/or sell products. Because we are listing them it does not mean we recommend them, or suggest that their products are suitable for you. Do carry out your own enquiries before buying or hiring any of the products offered by any of the organisations below. For independent advice speak to your midwife or health visitor.

Who to contact if you are worried about your own or your baby's health

- Contact your GP, health visitor or midwife.

NHS Direct
You can also contact NHS Direct for general health advice.
- Textphone users 18001 0845 606 4647 or 0845 606 4647
- Voice telephone users 0845 4647
- Website www.nhsdirect.nhs.uk

In an emergency
To call an ambulance:
Textphone users Dial 18000. This means you do not need to dial 999. Dialling 18000 on its own will give you a direct connection to the emergency services.
Voice telephone users Dial 999.

Contacting organisations by textphone
If you have a textphone and would like to contact organisations that don't have a textphone, you will need to use RNID Typetalk.

RNID Typetalk Customer Support
Telephone 0800 7311 888
Textphone 18001 0800 500 888
Fax 0151 709 8119
E-mail helpline@rnid-typetalk.org.uk
Website www.typetalk.org

General advice about pregnancy and childbirth

Ask your midwife, health visitor or GP for advice about getting pregnant, pregnancy, labour, birth and childcare.

www.babycentre.co.uk
A user-friendly and popular website for parents and parents-to-be.

www.baby-parenting.co.uk
A website full of information – from trying for a baby, to childbirth.

Midwives Information and Resource Service (MIDIRS)
An educational charity providing information and resources to midwives but with lots of useful information for parents. Ask for the Informed Choice Initiative pack of 15 leaflets.
MIDIRS, 9 Elmdale Road, Clifton,
Bristol BS8 1SL.
Telephone 0800 581 009
Website www.infochoice.org

National Childbirth Trust (NCT)
The National Childbirth Trust:
- Campaigns for better maternity care.
- Helps parents make friends with other new parents.
- Provides easy-to-read information.
- Provides free breastfeeding support.
- Runs antenatal classes in small groups and, in some cases, on a one-to-one basis.
The National Childbirth Trust,
Alexandra House, Oldham Terrace, Acton,
London W3 6NH.
Enquiries 0870 444 8707
Breastfeeding line 0870 444 8708
Textphone 020 8993 6714
Fax 0870 770 3237
E-mail
enquiries@national-childbirth-trust.co.uk
Website www.nctpregnancyandbabycare.com

WellBeing
WellBeing publishes a range of leaflets for women covering health in pregnancy.
Wellbeing, 27 Sussex Place,
Regents Park, London NW1 4SP.
Telephone 020 7772 6400
Fax 020 7724 7725
E-mail wellbeing@rcog.org.uk
Website www.wellbeing.org.uk

A-Z by topic

The rest of this section is arranged alphabetically (A-Z) into topics, for example, we start with information about *Antenatal tests* and end with information for *Working parents*.

Antenatal tests

ARC (Antenatal results and choices)
Support and information for parents throughout the antenatal testing process.
ARC, 73 Charlotte Street,
London W1T 4PN.
Helpline 020 7631 0285
Fax 020 7631 0280
E-mail info@arc-uk.org
Website www.arc-uk.org

Benefits for pregnant women and parents (see also *Working parents*)

Benefit Enquiry Line (BEL)
BEL is a free advice line run by the Department for Work and Pensions.
Telephone 0800 882200
Textphone 0800 243355
Northern Ireland: Telephone 0800 220674
Textphone 0800 243787

Maternity Alliance
Can give parents, and parents-to-be, advice about your rights at work and benefits you may be able to claim.
Maternity Alliance, Third Floor West, 2-6 Northburgh Street, London EC1V 0AY.
Information line 020 7490 7638
Fax 020 7014 1350
E-mail info@maternityalliance.org.uk
Website www.maternityalliance.org.uk

Childcare

www.childcarelink.gov.uk
Information on local and national childcare.

Daycare Trust
The Daycare Trust provides general information and advice about childcare.
Daycare Trust, 21 St George's Road,
London SE1 6ES.
Telephone 020 7840 3350
Fax 020 7840 3355
E-mail info@daycaretrust.org.uk
Website www.daycaretrust.org.uk

Communication services

Association of Lipspeakers (ALS)
For more information about lipreading and to book a lipspeaker.
ALS, 5 Furlong Close, Upper Tean,
Stoke-on-Trent ST10 4LB.
Telephone 01538 722482
Textphone 01538 722442
Fax 01538 722442
E-mail information@lipspeaking.co.uk
Website www.lipspeaking.co.uk

Council for the Advancement of Communication with Deaf People (CACDP)
CACDP has a directory that lists a range of human aids to communication, for example BSL/English interpreters, who are registered with CACDP.
CACDP, Durham University Science Park,
Block 4, Stockton Road,
Durham DH1 3UZ.
Telephone 0191 383 1155
Textphone 0191 383 7915
Fax 0191 383 7914
E-mail durham@cacdp.org.uk
Website www.cacdp.org.uk

RNID Information Line
The RNID Information Line can give you information about booking a communication service, including video interpreting.
RNID Information Line,
19-23 Featherstone Street,
London EC1Y 8SL.
Telephone 0808 808 0123
Textphone 0808 808 9000
Fax 020 7296 8199
E-mail informationline@rnid.org.uk
Website www.rnid.org.uk

Scottish Association of Sign Language Interpreters (SASLI)
If you need a BSL/English interpreter in Scotland, contact SASLI.
SASLI, Donaldson's College,
West Coates, Edinburgh EH12 5JJ.
Telephone 0131 347 5601
Textphone 0131 347 5601
Fax 0131 347 5628
E-mail mail@sasli.org.uk
Website www.sasli.org.uk

Wales Council for the Deaf
You can contact the Wales Council for the Deaf if you want to book a BSL/English interpreter in Wales.
Wales Council for the Deaf,
Glenview House, Courthouse Street,
Pontypridd CF37 1JY.
Telephone 01443 485687
Textphone 01443 485686
Fax 01443 408555
E-mail wcdeaf@freenet.co.uk
Website www.wcdeaf.org.uk

Complementary medicine

British Complementary Medicine Association
Can put you in touch with professional organisations to help you find a qualified practitioner.
British Complementary Medicine Association,
PO Box 5122,
Bournemouth, Dorset BH8 0WG.
Telephone 0845 345 5977
Fax 0845 345 5977
E-mail info@bcma.co.uk
Website www.bcma.co.uk

Institute for Complementary Medicine (ICM)
Contact the ICM if you would like to find a practitioner listed on the British Register of Complementary Medicine.
ICM, PO Box 194, London SE16 7QZ.
Telephone 020 7237 5165
Fax 020 7237 5175
E-mail icm@icmedicine.co.uk
Website www.icmedicine.co.uk

Cot deaths or Sudden infant death syndrome (SIDS)

The Foundation for the Study of Infant Deaths (FSID)
FSID can advise you on how to look after your baby safely and how to reduce the risk of a cot death.
FSID, Artillery House,
11-19 Artillery Row, London SW1P 1RT.
Helpline 0870 787 0554
Textphone 0870 787 0885
Fax 0870 787 0725
E-mail info@sids.org.uk
Website www.sids.org.uk/fsid/

Deaf and hard of hearing people (general information)

British Deaf Association (BDA)

The BDA Helpline provides a range of information and advice on subjects such as the Disability Discrimination Act (1995), welfare benefits, education, BSL and the Deaf community.
British Deaf Association,
1-3 Worship Street, London EC2A 2AB.
Helpline 0870 770 3300
Textphone 0800 652 2965
Videophone 020 7496 9539
Fax 020 7588 3527
E-mail helpline@bda.org.uk
Website www.bda.org.uk

Hearing Concern

Hearing Concern provides advice, support and information to hard of hearing adults. They also promote communication access and raise public and professional awareness of the issues associated with hearing loss.
Hearing Concern,
275/281 King Street, London W6 9LZ.
Helpdesk 0845 0744 600
Textphone 0845 0744 600
Fax 020 8742 9043
E-mail info@hearingconcern.org.uk
Website www.hearingconcern.org.uk

The National Deaf Children's Society (NDCS)

NDCS is an organisation of parents, families and carers. They provide information on audiology, communication, education, financial support and technology for deaf children. They also have a network of regional staff offering support near you, with special events for families.
NDCS, 15 Dufferin Street,
London EC1Y 8UR.
Freephone helpline 0808 800 8880
Textphone 0808 800 8880
Fax 0207 251 5020
E-mail helpline@ndcs.org.uk
Website www.ndcs.org.uk

RNID Information Line

The RNID Information Line offers a wide range of information on many aspects of being deaf or hard of hearing.
RNID Information Line,
19-23 Featherstone Street,
London EC1Y 8SL.
Telephone 0808 808 0123
Textphone 0808 808 9000
Fax 020 7296 8199
E-mail informationline@rnid.org.uk
Website www.rnid.org.uk

Deaf parenting

www.coda-international.org

A website for the adult, hearing children of deaf parents. CODA = Children of Deaf Adults.

www.deafparent.org.uk

A website specifically for deaf parents.

Deaf Parenting Project

Aims to raise awareness around issues of deaf parenting and improve services for deaf parents.
Contact DPPi for information (see later).

Deaf parenting e-mail group

An e-mail group that puts deaf parents, and professionals who work with them, in touch with each other to share information and offer support. Visit www.yahoogroups.com/groups/deafparenting or send a blank e-mail to deafparenting-subscribe@yahoogroups.com to join.

Local deaf parenting groups

Find out if there is a local group of deaf parents:
- Have a look on www.deafparent.org.uk
- Contact DPPi (see later).
- Contact your local council or social services to see if they are running a deaf parenting group.

Get in touch with other deaf mothers, with the National Childbirth Trust

The National Childbirth Trust has an **Experience register** that puts women in touch with other women to share experiences. If you would like to get in touch with other deaf mothers contact the Experience register:
Telephone 0870 444 8707
E-mail enquiries@national-childbirth-trust.co.uk

Disability Discrimination Act 1995 (DDA)

RNID Information Line

The RNID Information Line can send you a range of information on the Disability Discrimination Act (1995). See earlier for contact details.

RNID Casework Service

The RNID Casework Service provides information and advice to the public and professionals on the Disability Discrimination Act (1995). In some situations, the Casework Service may be able to help you bring your case to court, and provide you with representation in court.

RNID Casework Service,
19-23 Featherstone Street,
London EC1Y 8SL.
Telephone 0808 808 0123
Textphone 0808 808 9000
Fax 020 7296 8199
E-mail caseworkteam@rnid.org.uk

Citizens Advice Bureau (CAB)
Your local CAB will give free advice on the
Disability Discrimination Act (1995). In some
situations, they may provide representation. Do
an online search at www.citizensadvice.org.uk
or see your phonebook for your nearest CAB.

Community Legal Service
The Community Legal Service can give you
details of your local advice centre in England
and Wales.
Telephone 0845 608 1122
Textphone 0845 609 6677
Website www.justask.org.uk

The Disability Law Service (DLS)
The DLS provides free legal advice to disabled
people and representation where appropriate.
DLS, 39-45 Cavell Street, London E1 2BP.
Telephone 020 7791 9800
Textphone 020 7791 9801
Fax 020 7791 9802
E-mail advice@dls.org.uk
Website www.dls.org.uk

**The Disability Rights
Commission (DRC) Helpline**
The DRC provides free advice to people who
have been discriminated against. They may
also provide representation. They also run a
conciliation service to try and resolve problems
with service providers without going to court.
Disability Rights Commission,
Freepost MID 02164,
Stratford-upon-Avon CV37 9BR.
Telephone 08457 622 633
Textphone 08457 622 644
Fax 08457 778 878
E-mail enquiry@drc-gb.org
Website www.drc-gb.org

Law centres
The Law Centres Federation can give you the
details of your local law centre. Law centres
can provide free advice and representation.
Law Centres Federation,
18-19 Warren Street, London W1T 5LR.
Telephone 020 7387 8570
Fax 020 7387 8368
E-mail info@lawcentres.org.uk
Website www.lawcentres.org.uk

Patient Advocacy Liaison Service
Your local Patient Advocacy Liaison Service
can give you advice and support if you want to
make a complaint about hospital treatment.
Contact NHS Direct for more information. See
earlier for contact details.

Disabled children

BDF Newlife
Offers help to parents, carers and professionals
concerned about birth defects.
BDF Newlife, BDF Centre,
Hemlock Business Park, Hemlock Way,
Cannock WS11 7GF.
Telephone 01543 468888
Fax 01543 468999
Here to Help Nurse
Service 08700 70 70 20
Fax 01543 468999
E-mail info@bdfnewlife.co.uk
Website www.birthdefects.co.uk

Contact a Family
Information and support for families with
disabled children.
Contact a Family, 209-211 City Road,
London EC1V 1JN.
Contact a Family Helpline 0808 808 3555
Textphone 0808 803 3556
Fax 0207 608 8701
E-mail info@cafamily.org.uk
Website www.cafamily.org.uk

Mencap
Information and advice for people with
a learning disability, their families
and carers.
Mencap, 123 Golden Lane,
London EC1Y 0RT.
Telephone 0808 808 1111
Textphone 0808 8181
Fax 020 708 3254
E-mail help@mencap.org.uk
Website www.mencap.org.uk

Disabled parents

Disability, Pregnancy & Parenthood international (DPPi)

Contact DPPi for information and resources for disabled parents. They have information sheets about deaf parenting for deaf families and midwives. They also have a support worker for parents.
DPPi, National Centre for Disabled Parents,
Unit F9, 89-93 Fonthill Road, London N4 3JH.
Telephone 0800 018 4730
Textphone 0800 018 9949
Fax 020 7263 6399
E-mail info@dppi.org.uk
Website www.dppi.org.uk

Eating and drinking

Alcohol Concern

Visit www.alcoholconcern.org.uk for lots of information if you are concerned about your drinking.

Drinkline

Contact Drinkline if you are worried about your drinking during pregnancy.
Drinkline, Freepost, PO Box 4000,
Glasgow G3 8XX.
Telephone 0800 917 82 82
Textphone 0800 027 4114

Eating for pregnancy helpline

For advice on what to eat during pregnancy and while breastfeeding.
Eating for pregnancy helpline,
Centre for pregnancy nutrition,
University of Sheffield, Room 20,
The Jessop Wing, Tree Route Walk,
Sheffield S10 2SF.
Telephone 0845 130 3646
Fax 0114 226 1074
E-mail pregnancy.nutrition@sheffield.ac.uk
Website www.shef.ac.uk/pregnancy_nutrition

Equipment

www.rnid.org.uk/equipment

Database of equipment, such as baby monitors, and suppliers.

www.rnidshop.com

RNID Sound Advantage sells a range of equipment for deaf and hard of hearing people.

Feeding your baby

Association of Breastfeeding Mothers

The Association of Breastfeeding Mothers will put you in touch with a qualified breastfeeding counsellor if you need information or support. They also produce leaflets and booklets, which are useful for new parents.
The Association of Breastfeeding Mothers,
PO Box 207, Bridgwater TA6 7YT.
Helpline 020 7813 1481
Fax 01753 674766
E-mail info@abm.me.uk
Website www.abm.me.uk

www.breastfeeding.co.uk

Packed with information about breastfeeding.

The Breastfeeding Network

The Breastfeeding Network can give breastfeeding women support and information. Contact their Supporterline or drop in to one of their support centres and speak to a breastfeeding supporter face-to-face.
The Breastfeeding Network,
PO Box 11126, Paisley PA2 8YB.
Supporterline 0870 900 8787
E-mail email@breastfeedingnetwork.org.uk
Website www.breastfeedingnetwork.org.uk

La Leche League

La Leche League helps mothers to breastfeed. They give mother-to-mother support, encouragement, information and education. If you have an urgent enquiry you can contact their 24-hour helpline.
La Leche League (Great Britain),
PO Box 29, West Bridgford,
Nottingham NG2 7NP.
Helpline 0845 120 2918
Fax 0115 981 5597
E-mail enquiries@laleche.org.uk
Website www.lalecheleague.org

National Childbirth Trust (NCT)

The National Childbirth Trust supports all parents, however you feed your baby (see earlier for contact details). You can also contact their **Breastfeeding line** to speak to a trained counsellor if you are finding breastfeeding painful, or have any questions about breastfeeding.
Telephone 0870 444 8708
(Open 8am-10pm, every day of the year)

The UNICEF UK Baby Friendly Initiative

The Baby Friendly Initiative provides information about feeding and caring for your baby. This includes clear and easy-to-read leaflets on how to breastfeed successfully.
The UNICEF UK Baby Friendly Initiative, Africa House, 64-78 Kingsway,
London WC2B 6NB.
Telephone 020 7312 7652
Fax 020 7405 2332
E-mail bfi@unicef.org.uk
Website www.babyfriendly.org.uk

Immunisation/vaccination

www.immunisation.org.uk

A website which answers lots of questions about vaccinating your baby against diseases.

Labour and birth

Active Birth Centre

Information to help you make informed choices, and give you the confidence to be in charge of your pregnancy, birth and early parenting.
Active Birth Centre, 25 Bickerton Road,
London N19 5JT.
Telephone 020 7281 6760
Fax 020 7263 8098
E-mail info@activebirthcentre.com
Website www.activebirthcentre.com

The Association for Improvements in the Maternity Services (AIMS)

Advice and information about your choices and rights in maternity care.
AIMS, 5 Ann's Court, Grove Road,
Surbiton KT6 4BE.
Helpline 0870 765 1433
Fax 0870 765 1454
E-mail chair@aims.org.uk
Website www.aims.org.uk

www.babycaretens.co.uk

Information about the TENS machine for pain relief during labour, including where to hire one.

www.birthchoiceuk.com

A website to help you choose where to have your baby and who to help look after you in labour.

Independent Midwives Association

Information about finding and using an independent midwife.
Independent Midwives Association,
1 The Great Quarry, Guildford GU1 3XN.
Telephone 01483 821104
Website www.independentmidwives.org.uk

www.pulsar-tens.com

Information about the pulsar TENS machine for pain relief during labour.

Lone parents

Gingerbread

Support and advice for lone parents.
Gingerbread, 7 Sovereign Close, Sovereign Court, London E1W 3HW.
Telephone 0800 018 4318
Fax 020 7488 9333
E-mail membership@gingerbread.demon.co.uk
Website www.gingerbread.org.uk

One Parent Families

Information for lone parents on benefits, work, education, relationship breakdown, children and holidays.
One Parent Families,
255 Kentish Town Road,
London NW5 2LX.
Lone Parent Helpline 0800 018 5026
Fax 020 7482 4851
E-mail info@oneparentfamilies.org.uk
Website www.oneparentfamilies.org.uk

Meningitis

Meningitis Research Foundation

Information about meningitis including a subtitled video – *Holly's story*.
Meningitis Research Foundation,
Midland Way, Thornbury,
Bristol BS35 2BS.
Telephone 080 8800 3344
Fax 01454 281094
E-mail info@meningitis.org
Website www.meningitis.org

Miscarriage

Miscarriage Association

The Miscarriage Association can give you support and information if you have lost a baby during pregnancy.
Miscarriage Association, c/o Clayton Hospital, Northgate, Wakefield WF1 3JS.
Telephone 01924 200799
Fax 01924 298834
E-mail info@miscarriageassociation.org.uk
Website www.miscarriageassociation.org.uk

Newborn Hearing Screening

www.deafnessatbirth.org.uk
A website for professionals working with deaf children and their families, with lots of useful information for parents of deaf children.

National Deaf Children's Society (NDCS)
NDCS has a range of leaflets that explain the screening process.
See earlier for contact details.

Newborn Hearing Screening Programme
Information on the Newborn Hearing Screening programme in the UK including a BSL video with English subtitles. See the list of videos at the end of this section for more information.
E-mail nhsp@ihr.mrc.ac.uk
Website www.nhsp.info

New parents

Child Accident Prevention Trust
Information about how to help your child avoid accidents.
Child Accident Prevention Trust,
18-20 Farringdon Lane,
London EC1R 3HA.
Telephone 020 7608 3828
Fax 020 7608 3674
E-mail safe@capt.org.uk
Website www.capt.org.uk

Homestart
Information and support for families of children five years and under.
Homestart, 2 Salisbury Road,
Leicester LE1 7QR.
Helpline: 08000 68 63 68
Fax 0116 233 0232
E-mail info@home-start.org.uk
Website www.home-start.org.uk

Maternity Alliance
(See *Benefits* section earlier)

Parentline Plus
Help and information for anyone parenting a child.
Parentline Plus, 520 Highgate Studios,
53-79 Highgate Road, London NW5 1TL.
Helpline 0808 800 2222
Textphone 0800 783 6783
Fax 020 7284 5501
E-mail centraloffice@parentlineplus.org.uk
Website www.parentlineplus.org.uk

www.parentcentre.gov.uk
The Parent Centre is for all parents and carers who want to help their child or children to learn. It offers support, information and advice about your child's learning and the English education system.

Planning a baby

Foresight, The association for the promotion of preconceptual care
Information about how to make the most of your health, to make the most of your fertility.
Foresight, 28 The Paddock,
Godalming GU7 1XD.
Telephone 01483 427839
Fax 01483 427668
E-mail foresighthq@btopenworld.com
Website
www.foresight-preconception.org.uk

Human Fertilisation and Embryology Authority
Advice if you are thinking about having treatment to help you get pregnant.
Human Fertilisation and Embryology Authority,
Paxton House,
30 Artillery Lane, London E1 7LS.
Telephone 0207 377 5077
Fax 0207 377 1871
E-mail admin@hfea.gov.uk
Website www.hfea.gov.uk

Postnatal depression

Association for Post-Natal Illness
Support for mothers who have postnatal illness.
The Association for Post-Natal Illness,
145 Dawes Road, Fulham,
London SW6 7EB.
Helpline 020 7386 0868
Fax 020 7386 8885
E-mail info@apni.org
Website www.apni.org

Pre-eclampsia

Action on Pre-eclampsia (APEC)
Information to help you understand and care for this condition.
Action on Pre-eclampsia,
84-88 Pinner Road, Harrow HA1 4HZ.
Helpline 020 8427 4217
Fax 020 8424 0653
E-mail enquiries@apec.org.uk
Website www.apec.org.uk

Smoking

Quit
Information and support to help you and your partner stop smoking.
Quit, 211 Old Street, London EC1V 9NR.
Quitline 0800 00 22 00
Textphone 0800 00 22 22
Fax 0207 251 1661
E-mail stopsmoking@quit.org.uk
Website www.quit.org.uk

NHS Pregnancy Smoking Helpline
Advice and support to help you stop smoking.
Telephone 0800 169 0 169
Website www.givingupsmoking.co.uk

Social services

Family Rights Group
Advice and support for families whose children are involved with social services.
Family Rights Group, The Print House,
18 Ashwin Street, London E8 3DL.
Telephone advice line 0800 731 1696
Fax 020 7923 2683
E-mail advice@frg.org.uk
Website www.frg.org.uk

Special care babies

BLISS – the premature baby charity
Provides support and information to parents and families who have, or have had, a baby in special care.
BLISS – the premature baby charity,
68 South Lambeth Road,
London SW8 1RL.
Telephone 0870 770 0337
Fax 0870 770 0338
E-mail information@bliss.org.uk
Website www.bliss.org.uk

Stillbirth

Stillbirth and Neonatal Death Society (SANDS)
Supports parents and their families who have experienced the death of a baby before, during, or shortly after birth. Also has local support groups, literature and a telephone helpline.
SANDS, 28 Portland Place,
London W1B 1LY.
Helpline 020 7436 5881
Fax 020 7436 3715
E-mail support@uk-sands.org
Website www.uk-sands.org

Twins and multiple births

Tamba
Information and support for families of twins, triplets and more.
Tamba, 2 The Willows, Gardner Road,
Guildford GU1 4PG.
Telephone 0800 138 0509
Fax 0870 770 3303
E-mail enquiries@tamba.org.uk
Website www.tamba.org.uk

Unplanned pregnancy

Family planning clinic
Check your local telephone directory for details of your local clinic or ask your GP.

Marie Stopes International
Can give you information on a range of sexual health issues including contraception and abortion.
Marie Stopes International,
153-157 Cleveland Street,
London W1T 6QW.
Telephone 020 7574 7400
Fax 020 7574 7417
Website www.mariestopes.org.uk

Working parents – maternity and paternity rights (see also *Benefits* earlier)

www.dti.gov.uk
A government website with information about rights for working parents.

Jobcentre Plus
Advice about making a claim for Maternity Allowance or Incapacity Benefit.
See your phone book or visit www.jobcentreplus.gov.uk for contact details of your local office.

Maternity Alliance
See *Benefits* section earlier.

www.tiger.gov.uk
A user-friendly guide to employment law.

Trade union
If you are a member of a trade union ask your representative for advice at work.

Working families

Information for working families including a support network for parents of children with disabilities.

Working families, 1-3 Berry Street, London EC1V 0AA.

Helpline 0800 013 0313

Fax 020 7253 6253

E-mail office@workingfamilies.org.uk

Website www.workingfamilies.org.uk

Useful reading

Most of the organisations listed in this chapter will have free or low-cost leaflets and books. Have a look at their website or send off for a list of their publications. We have also included some books, leaflets and videos that have been particularly recommended by parents interviewed for this book and members of the book's advisory panel.

Change publications

You can get the following publications from Change. They use lots of pictures and very little writing.

• *Depo-Provera.*
• *Planning a baby.*
• *You and your baby. 0 to 1.*

All are available from:

Change, Units 19 and 20,

Unity Business Centre,

26 Roundhay Road, Leeds LS7 1AB.

Telephone 0113 243 0202

Textphone 0113 243 2225

Fax 0113 243 0220

E-mail change.north@tesco.net

Website www.changepeople.co.uk

Department of Health publications

You can get a range of publications from the Department of Health.

• *Consent – what you have a right to expect, a guide for parents.*
• *How to bottle feed.*
• *How to breastfeed.*
• *The Pregnancy Book. 2001.*
  This book is given free to all first time mothers in England but you can also buy it if you contact the Department of Health.

All are available from the Department of Health.

Telephone 08701 555 455

Textphone 01623 756236

Fax 01623 724524

E-mail doh@prolog.uk.com

Website www.doh.gov.uk

DPPi publications

DPPi publishes a range of plain English factsheets for deaf parents.

• *Antenatal appointments.*
• *Deaf families – information for deaf and hard of hearing parents.*
• *Deaf parent and family groups.*
• *Labour.*
• *The maternity ward.*

All are available from DPPi (see *Disabled parents* section earlier for contact details).

National Childbirth Trust publications

The National Childbirth Trust publishes a complete range of books about pregnancy, childbirth and parenting, including:

• *Complete Book Of Pregnancy.* NCT National Childbirth Trust. 2000. (Thorsons in collaboration with National Childbirth Trust Publishing).
• *Feelings after Birth. The NCT book of Postnatal Depression.* Heather Welford. 2002. (National Childbirth Trust Publishing).

All are available from the National Childbirth Trust Maternity Sales.

Telephone 0870 112 1120

Website www.nctms.co.uk

RNID publications

RNID publishes a wide range of information for deaf and hard of hearing people. The following factsheets may be of particular interest to deaf parents and parents-to-be:

• *Baby monitors – information for deaf and hard of hearing people.* 2003.
• *The Disability Discrimination Act (1995) (DDA) – a guide for deaf and hard of hearing customers.* 2003.
• *Genetics and deafness.* 2004.
• *The Human Rights Act 1998 – information for deaf and hard of hearing people.* 2003.
• *Middle ear conditions.* 2003.
• *Newborn Hearing Screening.* 2003.

All are available from the RNID Information Line (see *Deaf and Hard of Hearing people* section for contact details).

Other publications

- *Life After Birth.* Kate Figes. 2000. (Penguin).
- *Annabel Karmel's Complete First Year Planner: In association with Great Ormond Street Hospital.* Annabel Karmel. 2003. (Ebury Press).
- *Pregnancy Question and Answer book.* Dr Christopher Lees, Dr Karina Reynolds and Grainne McCartan. 2002. (Dorling Kindersley).
- *Your Child at Play – Birth to One Year. Discovering the Senses and Learning About the World.* Marilyn Segal, Wendy Masi. 2000. (Vermilion).
- *First-time parents.* Dr Miriam Stoppard. 2001. (Dorling Kindersley).

Videos

- *Deaf parents – gaps in services.* 2002. BSL with English subtitles. This video shows deaf parents sharing their experiences of maternity services in the UK. 2002. (Available from DPPi, see *Disabled parents* section earlier).
- *The Disability Discrimination Act (DDA).* 2003. *The DDA and your rights.* BSL with English subtitles. (Available from RNID see *Deaf and hard of hearing people* section earlier).
- *Holly's story.* 2003. English subtitles. Information about meningitis. (Available from the Meningitis Research Foundation, see *Meningitis* section earlier).
- *NHS Newborn Screening Programme.* 2003. BSL with English subtitles and voice over. Free loan to pregnant women in areas with a Newborn Hearing Screening Programme. Ask your midwife for a free copy. To buy a copy contact the Newborn Hearing Screening Programme (see *Newborn Hearing Screening* section earlier).

Glossary

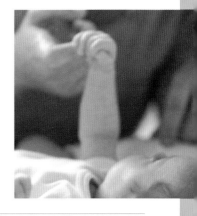

Over the next few pages we have listed medical words and terms that we have used in this book, along with a description of what they mean. You may also find it useful to have a look at our diagram in *Chapter 2 Planning a baby* for more information. You will also find more information throughout this book.

Afterbirth
(see placenta below)

Amniocentesis
A test which is usually done at around 20 weeks of pregnancy. It is used to tell whether your baby has a condition such as Down's syndrome.

Amniotic fluid
When your baby is in the womb she floats in a fluid known as the amniotic fluid. It is also known as 'waters'.

Antenatal
The time you are pregnant, before giving birth.

Areola
The darker skin around your nipple.

Caesarean section or
Caesarean birth
A caesarean section is an operation to help deliver your baby.

Cervix
The opening to your womb at the top of your vagina. It is usually closed but when you are in labour it opens (dilates) till it is about 10cm wide.

Chorionic villus sampling (CVS)
This is a test that may be offered to women before they are 14 weeks pregnant. This test will be able to tell definitely whether your baby has a condition such as Down's syndrome or another genetic condition.

Chromosomes
Genes provide our bodies with the information they need to grow and function. They are stored in chromosomes. Every cell in your body, or your baby's body, contains 23 pairs of chromosomes.

Contractions
One of the signs that you are in labour. This is when your womb tightens up and then lets go. Contractions gradually get stronger and more frequent as your labour goes on.

Down's syndrome
People with Down's syndrome have learning difficulties and may have heart and lung problems. However, many can go on to lead independent adult lives with some support.

Doula
A woman who has learned how to give particular support to women when they give birth.

Ectopic pregnancy

An ectopic pregnancy is when a fertilised egg starts growing outside the womb, generally in the fallopian tube.

Embryo

Embryo is the word used to describe a baby up to the beginning of the third month of pregnancy. After that it's known as a foetus.

Epidural

An epidural is when a drug – a local anaesthetic – is injected into a space around your spinal cord. It stops you feeling anything from the waist down including the pain of your contractions. It may also make it difficult for you to move from the waist down.

Episiotomy

A cut made through the back wall of the vagina into the perineum (see *perineum* below), to make it easier for your baby to be born.

Fallopian tube

Tubes that link your ovaries to your womb.

Foetus

The name given to a baby after the beginning of the third month of pregnancy.

Folic acid

A vitamin that helps prevent your baby being born with conditions such as spina bifida.

Forceps

Forceps look like stainless steel salad servers. Doctors may use them to help deliver your baby.

General anaesthetic

A drug which you are given to make you lose feeling and reduce pain. If you have a general anaesthetic you are not awake.

Gynaecologist

A doctor specialising in the care and treatment of women who have problems with their reproductive system.

Heartburn

Heartburn is an unpleasant burning feeling that you feel behind your breastbone. Some women develop it during pregnancy.

Hormones

Chemicals which your body produces and which lead to changes in your body.

Immunisation

A way of protecting your baby against serious diseases.

Induced birth

An induced birth means you are given help to start your labour.

Lanugo

Downy hair which covers your baby when she is in the womb.

Local anaesthetic

A drug, which you are given to help you lose feeling and reduce pain in a particular part of your body. If you have a local anaesthetic, you stay awake.

Lochia

After birth you will lose some blood through your vagina. This can go on for several weeks. It comes from your womb – where the placenta was attached to the inside of the womb.

Meconium

A thick, sticky, greenish black substance which your baby will poo in the few days after she is born.

Miscarriage

If you lose a baby in the first 24 weeks of pregnancy this is known as a miscarriage. A miscarriage is also sometimes called a 'spontaneous abortion'.

Morning sickness

Morning sickness is also known as pregnancy sickness. You can feel sick at different times in the day and not just in the morning. You may only feel a little bit sick or you may feel sick every day and may actually vomit.

Nuchal fold

A pad of skin at the back of your baby's neck which can be measured when your baby is in the womb. This is used for testing for conditions such as Down's syndrome.

Obstetrician

A doctor specialising in the care and treatment of women planning to get pregnant, during their pregnancy and after they have given birth.

Ovary/ovaries

Women have two ovaries. They are joined to your fallopian tubes and produce your eggs.

Over-the-counter medicine

Medicine that you can buy 'over-the-counter' at the pharmacist, without having to see your GP first. **Always tell your pharmacist you are pregnant and ask for advice before buying any over-the-counter medicine.**

Paediatrician

A doctor specialising in the medical treatment and care of children.

Perineum

The area of your body that stretches between the back of your vagina to your anus.

Pessary

A pessary is medicine that you put in your vagina, for example, your GP or pharmacist might suggest you use a pessary if you have thrush. **Always tell your pharmacist you are pregnant and ask for advice before buying any over-the-counter medicine.**

Placenta

The placenta is also called the afterbirth. It forms in the womb when you are pregnant. It allows your baby to get all its oxygen and food from you.

Postnatal

The time after you have given birth to your baby.

A show

One of the signs you may be in labour. This is when the plug of mucous that has formed in the neck of your womb, comes away. It will look like clear jelly or may be pink or red if it is stained with blood.

Spina bifida

A condition which affects your baby's spine leading to nerve damage. People with spina bifida can be paralysed from the waist down or they may have very few symptoms.

TENS

TENS = transcutaneous electrical nerve stimulation. A TENS machine gives out small pulses that block the pain messages being sent to the brain during labour and encourages your body to produce endorphins.

Thrush

Thrush is a thick, itchy white discharge from your vagina. It is also known as candida or yeast infection.

Umbilical cord

The cord which links your baby to your placenta when your baby is in the womb.

Ultrasound scan

An ultrasound scan allows you to see what your baby looks like when she is lying in your womb. You will see this picture on what looks like a television screen.

Uterus

Another word for the womb. See *womb* below.

Vagina

The passage between your cervix and your vulva. Your baby will travel from your womb and down your vagina when she is born.

Varicose veins

These are veins in your leg or bottom that can become bigger and more painful during pregnancy.

Ventouse

Doctors may use a ventouse to help deliver your baby. It looks like a small plastic cup and is attached to a vacuum. Suction is used to help the cup stick to your baby's head and to help pull your baby out.

Vernix

The name of the protective coating which covers your baby in your womb starting when you are about five months pregnant.

Vulva

The outer part of the vagina (the part you can see). Your baby travels down your vagina and through your vulva when she is born.

Waters breaking

This is one of the signs that you may be in labour. The 'waters' is the word given to the liquid that surrounds your baby in the womb. Waters don't always break at the start of labour. If they do, they may gush out or just be a trickle.

Womb

The womb is also known as the uterus. This is where your baby will live and grow during your pregnancy.

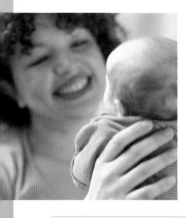

Index

RNID Publications
catalogue

Out now with over 150 publications, videos, CD ROMS, cassettes and CDs on being deaf, tinnitus, hearing aids, technology and much more.

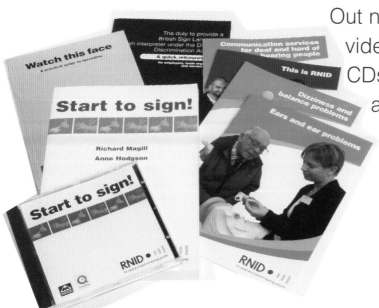

To order your free copy, contact:
RNID Information Line,
19-23 Featherstone Street,
London EC1Y 8SL
Telephone 0808 808 0123
Textphone 0808 808 9000
Fax 020 7296 8199
E-mail informationline@rnid.org.uk
Website www.rnid.org.uk

The RNID Information Line

The RNID Information Line is a good place to start if you want information on many aspects of being deaf or hard of hearing, or about the work we do. Here are just a few of the questions we are able to help with:

• Where can I get a baby monitor for deaf people?
• What is the DDA?
• Can you tell me more about the Human Rights Act?
• What is Newborn Hearing Screening?
• How do I book a BSL/English interpreter?

RNID Information Line,
19-23 Featherstone Street, London EC1Y 8SL
Telephone 0808 808 0123
Textphone 0808 808 9000
Fax 020 7296 8199
E-mail informationline@rnid.org.uk
Website www.rnid.org.uk

www.rnid.org.uk

Our website is a great source of information.
• Download our free factsheets and leaflets.
• See what's new in technology.
• Buy equipment and books in the RNID shop.
• Join our discussion forum.
• View video clips of signs to help you practise your BSL.

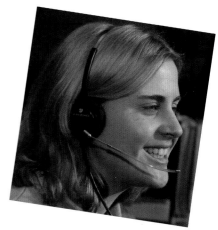

Have you seen the **new**

A step in the right direction **Solutions catalogue?**

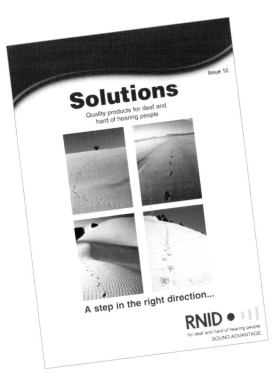

Over 150 products, including baby monitors, to help with a variety of hearing losses.

To receive your FREE copy call

Customer Service Team
Telephone **0870 789 8855**
Textphone **01733 238020**
or order online at **www.rnidshop.com**

Membership - get connected

The information and advice that you have received in this book does not stop here. Joining the other 34,000 RNID members is an excellent way of receiving up-to-date information on deafness, hearing loss and tinnitus as well as our influential campaigns. All members benefit from:

- **One in Seven**, our information packed bi-monthly magazine.

- **10% off** RNID priced publications.

- A **£5 voucher** towards equipment from RNID Sound Advantage.

- Access to **RNID Select** – special offers on a range of leading brands.

- Being part of the **campaign** to improve the lives of deaf and hard of hearing people.

How to **join**

Membership is open to all and costs £19.50 per year, or only £12.50 if you are retired, unwaged or a full time student.
It's easy to join:

Visit **www.rnid.org.uk/join** or

Call **0845 634 0679** (telephone/textphone) for an application form.

You can save £2 off the standard price of membership by paying by Direct Debit. Contact the Membership Helpline on telephone/textphone 0845 634 0679 for information.

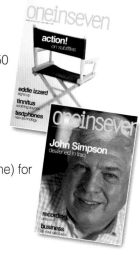

Get connected and **join today!**

RNID typetalk

Helping everyone use the phone

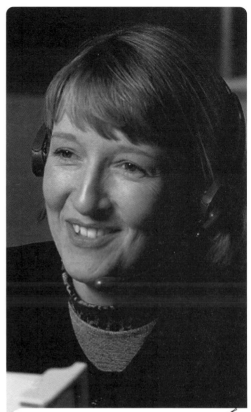

Did you know, even if you have lost your hearing or your voice you can still use the telephone?

RNID Typetalk is the only national telephone relay service for deaf, deafened, deafblind, hard of hearing and speech-impaired people.

Making a call through RNID Typetalk is just like making a standard telephone call.
You can have a full, real-time conversation, unlike SMS text messaging where you have to wait for the next part of the message.

RNID Typetalk is free to use and is available 24 hours a day, seven days a week.

For more information visit our website at **www.typetalk.org** or call our Customer Support Team free on:
Telephone 0800 7311 888 **Textphone** 18001 0800 500 888
(Monday to Friday 8am-8pm. Weekends 9am-5pm)

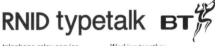

RNID typetalk **BT**
telephone relay service   *Working together*

---

have you ever thought of helping with
RNID's work?

Well, this is your opportunity to raise not only money but much needed awareness too.

Here are just a few ways that you can help:

- Make a donation – you can give on a regular basis, or make a one-off gift.

- Become a volunteer – we are always looking for people willing to give up their time.

- Support our campaigning work. For example, we are working hard to secure the rollout of newborn hearing screening across the UK.

- Fundraise at work, with friends, or with any group you're involved in.

For more information please contact
Supporter Services
Telephone 020 7296 8264
Textphone 020 7296 8264 **Fax** 020 7296 8129
E-mail supporterservices@rnid.org.uk

There is a whole range of ways you can support RNID. If you would like more information about any of the ideas here, or have any of your own, please do not hesitate to contact us or visit our website at www.rnid.org.uk

It is only with the support of people like you that we can continue our vital work. Thank you.

Introducing the National Childbirth Trust

The UK's biggest support group for parents-to-be and new parents

Help – you're pregnant for the first time, you know nothing about birth or babies... Next thing, you have a newborn baby in your arms and you've never even changed a nappy in your life before!

That's where The National Childbirth Trust comes in.

Who better to help you with the whole upheaval of pregnancy, birth and a new baby than a network of other women and men who've just been through it all and know how hard it can be?

Run by parents, for parents, The National Childbirth Trust (NCT) is a self-help charity that covers the UK. There's bound to be a local branch near you, running
- childbirth classes
- new baby groups
- open house get-togethers
- support for dads
- nearly new sales of baby clothes and equipment
  – as well as loads of other events where you can meet other people going through the same changes.

Preparing for a baby
There's a lot to learn about birth and life with a newborn. Trained NCT antenatal teachers are there to help. Both you and your partner (or whoever plans to be with you at the birth) are welcome at our antenatal classes. You'll meet others at the same stage of pregnancy and learn a lot. To find out how to book classes telephone 0870 444 8707, textphone 020 8993 6713 or visit www.nctpregnancyandbabycare.com

Getting bigger?
Bras that were comfortable before pregnancy become unbearable. We have a range of best-selling bras for pregnancy and breastfeeding. Telephone 0870 112 1120 for our free catalogue. It contains lots of books, toys, baby goods and gifts, too. And you can also order online at www.nctms.co.uk

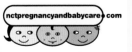

NCT information website
Next time you log on to the Internet, look at our website. It's got loads of information on pregnancy, labour, birth, breastfeeding, babycare and toddler development. You'll also be able to post your own questions on the site and get personal replies.

But we can't afford a baby!
That's what our famous Nearly New Sales are for – helping new parents make ends meet by offering high-quality baby items at knockdown prices. If you look at our website (see previous column), and click on NEWS on the home page, you'll find upcoming sales listed, all full of bargains.

Life after birth
And if you want to meet other mums and dads, to talk about the change that a new baby has made to your lives – ask about our postnatal courses or drop-ins. They're very popular.

New to breastfeeding?
We offer free help with breastfeeding if you're finding it difficult. Our award-winning NCT breastfeeding telephone line has now been going for nearly two years. Give one of our breastfeeding counsellors a call on telephone 0870 444 8708. 8am–10pm.

What's on where?
Suddenly you need to know where to go with a baby! Your local NCT newsletter is a useful source of information. There are all sorts of places and events in your area that you did not know existed before you became parents. To be sure of a copy, join the NCT by contacting our membership hotline (see below).

Become a member for £36
NCT services and support are open to everyone. We encourage people to join the charity so that you can help fund our work – supporting other new parents like you.

Want to know more about the NCT before you join? Telephone 0870 444 8707 or textphone 020 8993 6714 and we'll send you an information pack.

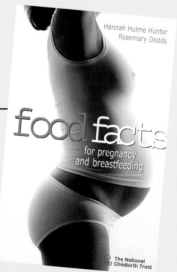